human hair *diversity*

DR JOHN GRAY

All that we are is determined by our genes.

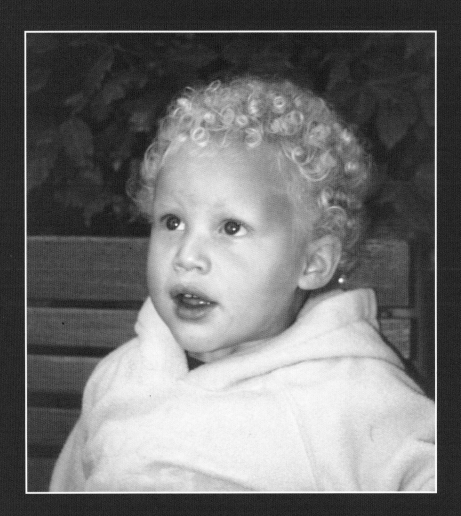

The hair of this
brown-eyed Nordic child is
the result of an unusual
combination of genes. The
genes of the cells of the
hair follicle, which
regulate the proteins that
form the hair shaft, have
here produced
uncharacteristic but
spectacular light, tight
curls.
All of us are linked by
genes that derive from a
single region of the world.

human hair *diversity*

WRITTEN AND PHOTOGRAPHED BY
D R   J O H N   G R A Y

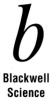

**Blackwell
Science**

© 2000 by
Dr John Gray

Published by Blackwell Science Ltd.

Editorial Offices:
Osney Mead, Oxford OX2 0EL
25 John Street, London WC1N 2BL
23 Ainslie Place, Edinburgh EH3 6AJ
350 Main Street, Malden, MA 02148 5018, USA
54 University Street, Carlton,
Victoria 3053, Australia
10, rue Casimir Delavigne, 75006 Paris, France

Other Editorial Offices:
Blackwell Wissenschafts-Verlag GmbH
Kurfürstendamm 57, 10707 Berlin, Germany

Blackwell Science KK
MG Kodenmacho Building, 7–10 Kodenmacho
Nihombashi, Chuo-ku, Tokyo 104, Japan

The right of the author to be identified as the
Author of this Work has been asserted in
accordance with the Copyright, Designs and
Patents Act 1988.

First published 2000.

Printed in Great Britain by The Alden Group,
Oxford.

Designed and set by Em Quad.

The Blackwell Science logo is a trade mark of
Blackwell Science Ltd, registered at the United
Kingdom Trade Marks Registry

DISTRIBUTORS
Marston Book Services Ltd
PO Box 269
Abingdon
Oxon OX14 4YN
ORDERS:
Tel: 01235 465500
Fax: 01235 465555

USA
Blackwell Science, Inc.
Commerce Place
350 Main Street,
Malden, MA 02148 5018
ORDERS:
Tel: 800-759-6012
     781-388-8250
Fax: 781-388-8255

Canada
Login Brothers Book Company
324 Saulteaux Crescent
Winnipeg, Manitoba R3J 3T2
Canada, L4W 4P7
ORDERS:
Tel: 204-837-2987

Australia
Blackwell Science Pty Ltd
54 University Street
Carlton, Victoria 3053
ORDERS:
Tel: 3-9347-0300
Fax: 3-9347-5001

A catalogue record for this title is available from
the British Library

ISBN: 0 632 05672 X

For further information on Blackwell Science,
visit our website:
www.blackwell-science.com

Contents

The author

Dr John Gray is a general practitioner who has a long-standing interest in skin and hair problems. He is a member of the European and American Hair Research Societies and of the Royal Society of Medicine. He is a consultant to Procter & Gamble and is involved in their hair education programme, and has lectured widely on the subject of hair health to doctors and hairdressers.

Acknowledgements

The author would like to express his thanks to the following:

Professor Chris Stringer, Head of Human Origins at The Natural History Museum, London, for his advice and counsel in developing this publication

Dorte and Kristiana, for helping me genuinely understand the psychology of hair and 'hair care'

Hair Collections Club, Weybridge, Surrey

Terry Jacques Salon, Clapham, London

Jean Macqueen, my most splendid editor

Chris Gummer, Senior Research Fellow — Procter & Gamble, for his encouragement and help

Janet Smith, my long-suffering secretary for her help in organising this book

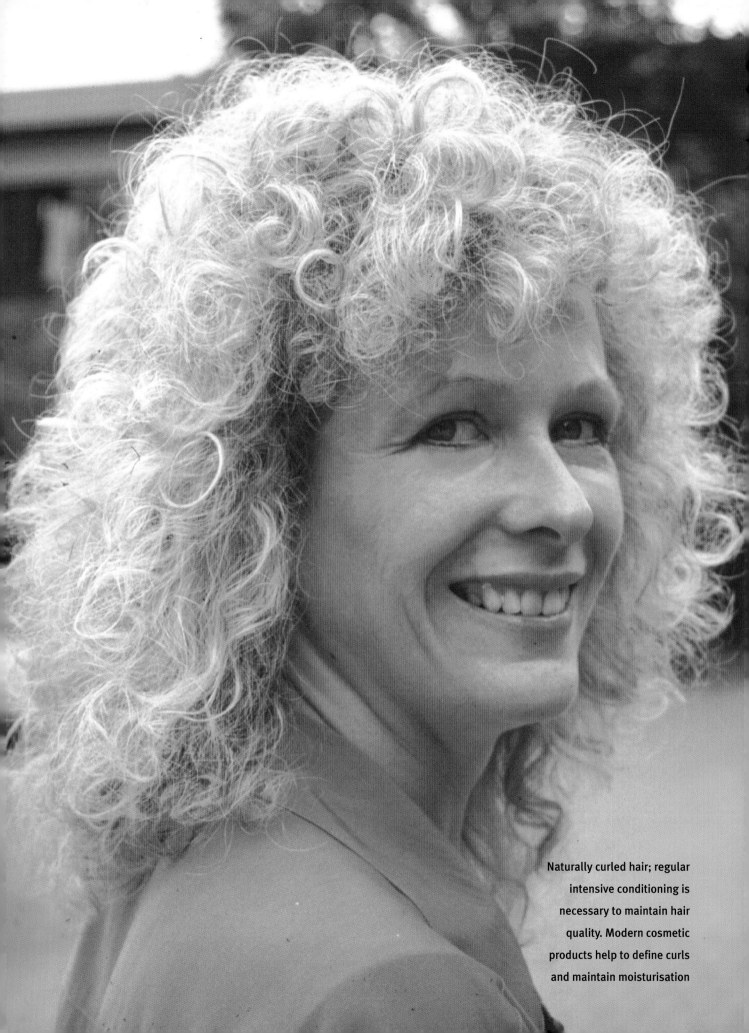

Naturally curled hair; regular intensive conditioning is necessary to maintain hair quality. Modern cosmetic products help to define curls and maintain moisturisation

Introduction

Scalp hair is perhaps the single most distinctive feature that an individual bears. If we humans had evolved as a totally hairless species (a rarity among mammals), we would probably form a far more apparently homogeneous population than the diversity we see in the world around us.

Each one of us, even if we have an identical twin, is genetically unique. Each is separated from the other six billion people on the Earth by differences – some of them obvious, others almost indiscernible without elaborate chemical analysis – derived from their genetic 'print'. Our fingerprints tell of this uniqueness. Our hair, although less obviously, may be such a 'fingerprint' – a visible expression of both our individuality and our diversity. Through our scalp hair, which is an important display signal at distance, and through the dissemination of sexual scents associated with the hair in intimate areas of the body, we find a means of asserting our identity.

If an individual suddenly loses a significant amount of hair, the appearance is radically altered: he or she may become unrecognisable. Imagine, for a moment, a world in which everyone lacked such adornment. Consider the contributions of the form and style of hair to such 20th-century icons as Marilyn Monroe, Albert Einstein, Princess Diana, Bob Marley and even current and past political leaders.

Yet whatever hair 'nature' has given us, many of us seek to change or enhance some feature of it, even going so far as to mimic hair that is far removed in appearance from our own, whether in colour, or style, or form. Today individuals seek to

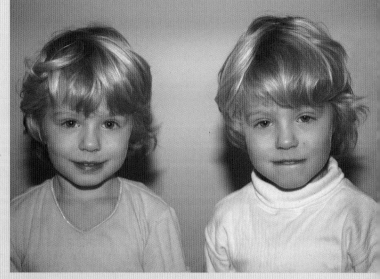

Identical twins inherit the same genes from their parents, including the genes for their hair form.

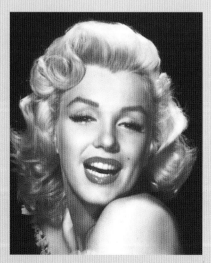

The supreme platinum blonde icon!

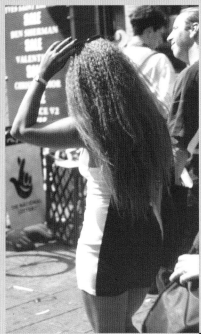

create a hair 'style' to represent their 'image', define their position in society, express rebellion or simply cope. How an understanding of the unique properties of our hair can allow us to achieve what is increasingly termed 'end benefit' is part of this discussion.

In the past, scientists tended to describe the anatomy of the hair shaft with reference to 'race' or 'ethnic' background. On this basis it is easy to create an over-simplistic approach to hair, particularly in respect of its cosmetic potential. Reality is far more complex. Tightly curled hair like that of peoples originating from sub-Saharan Africa, and their descendants, is occasionally seen in light-skinned Indo-Europeans. Similarly the thick, dark resilient hair characteristic of many Oriental Asians can appear in people from other parts of the world.

Individuals who have chosen to make dramatic changes in their hair form and colour: naturally dark Afro-Caribbean and black Thai hair (above and right respectively) have both undergone radical transformation from their natural form and colour.

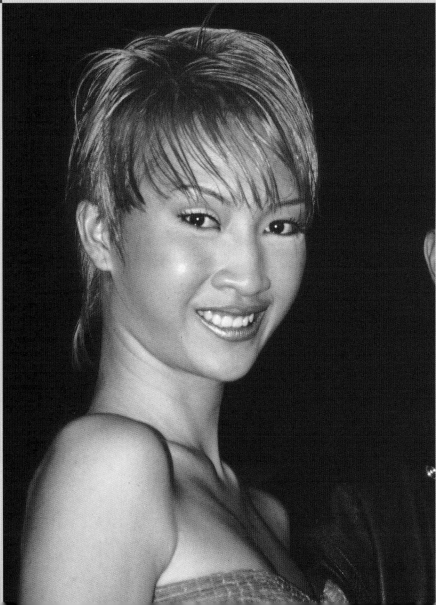

The constant movement of genes within the increasingly mobile human population inexorably tends to homogenisation of the human species but, curiously, the result may be an increase in individual diversity. On a global basis, human variation seen in terms of 'race' may eventually be deemed irrelevant other than as local limitations of universal human traits.

Why is there such profound diversity in this one particular aspect of our appearance? There is no simple answer to such a question. The development of a scientific understanding of the evolution of human hair diversity is hampered by the scantiness of fossil and archaeological records of hair. At the time of writing, however, the entire genetic makeup of the human species is undergoing intense study, and the results of this work may ultimately lead to a deeper understanding of the mystery.

We do know that within the human evolutionary process, certain genetic characteristics were important. One example is the resistance to malaria possessed by people who carry the gene that makes them susceptible to sickle cell anaemia. In both Africa and the Mediterranean region there are populations that carry these protective genes, but they do not necessarily coincide with any one recognised 'racial' group. There is little evidence for hair form being associated with disease resistance.

What then is the evolutionary advantage, if any, of such an attribute as a 'head of hair'? It has been suggested that scalp hair evolved to protect the scalp from the harmful effects of sunlight, or to conserve body heat, or even as a defence against insects! This is not supported by physiological evidence, however. The probability is that scalp hair in both sexes, and possibly also facial hair in men, is associated with only one major activity: sex, or more precisely mate selection.

Every individual's potential hair form is determined at the time of conception. Until it naturally or prematurely departs we consciously or subconsciously use it as part of our daily lives. People care for this asset (fortunately, for most of us, a renewable one – see box on page 5) in a manner that varies from the obsessional to the scandalously negligent.

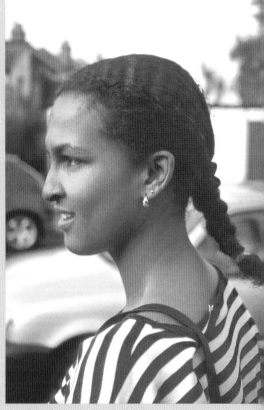

This lady originates from north-eastern Africa. Her hair is naturally wavy rather than tightly curled – this may be the 'African Eve'.

Brilliant naturally red hair with almost Oriental form from north-western Europe. The evolutionary significance of red hair is as yet unknown.

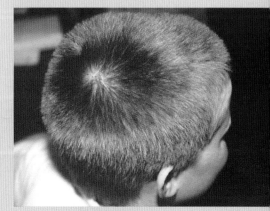

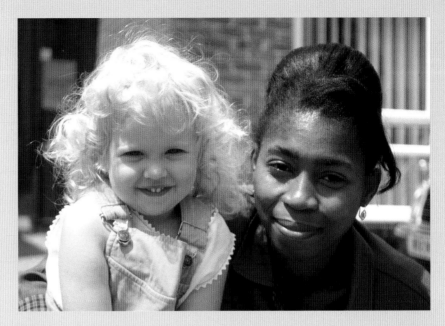

The range of human diversity is vast This African lady has 'relaxed' her hair.

An understanding of the structure and physical properties of our hair allows us to assess realistically what its aesthetic capabilities and limitations may be. In the evolution of hair as a sexual signal, adornment and status statement, these individual limitations will permit only certain variations of style without gross effects on the hair structure. It is the joint roles of the cosmetic scientist, the product formulator and the hair stylist, expertly exploiting their understanding, to help us meet our needs as individuals surrounded by a sea of diversity.

Facial hair as well as scalp hair is probably only associated with sexual attraction.

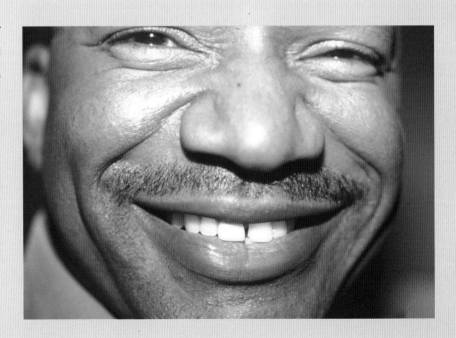

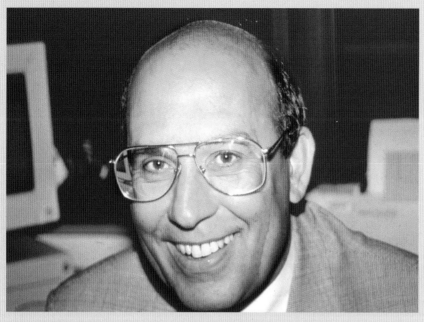

Androgenetic alopecia in humans is part of our genetic inheritance.

Our expectations of hair's aesthetic possibilities
are sometimes founded more in hope than reality!

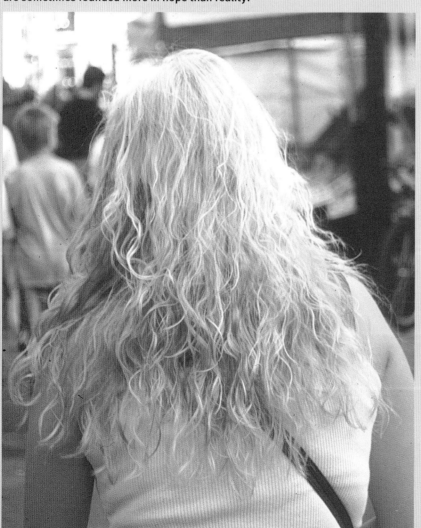

THE SIGNIFICANCE OF HAIR LOSS

It has been suggested that our primate relatives who display balding characteristics in both sexes illustrate a stage in an evolutionary trend where scalp signals are related to 'power' and 'status', while body hair differences are part of mating signals.

There are geographical as well as age-related differences in the incidence or pattern of hair loss in male androgenetic alopecia. African-American, Asian and Native American men tend to have less extensive baldness than Indo-Europeans.

Balding is a complex genetically inherited disorder that increases with ageing and is probably under the effects of male hormones (androgens). One-quarter of all males at age 25 show signs of androgenetic alopecia, a figure that rises to one-half at age 50.

It has recently been suggested that this balding trend may even be in the process of being reversed in humans. It is not clear whether this is true for female pattern baldness.

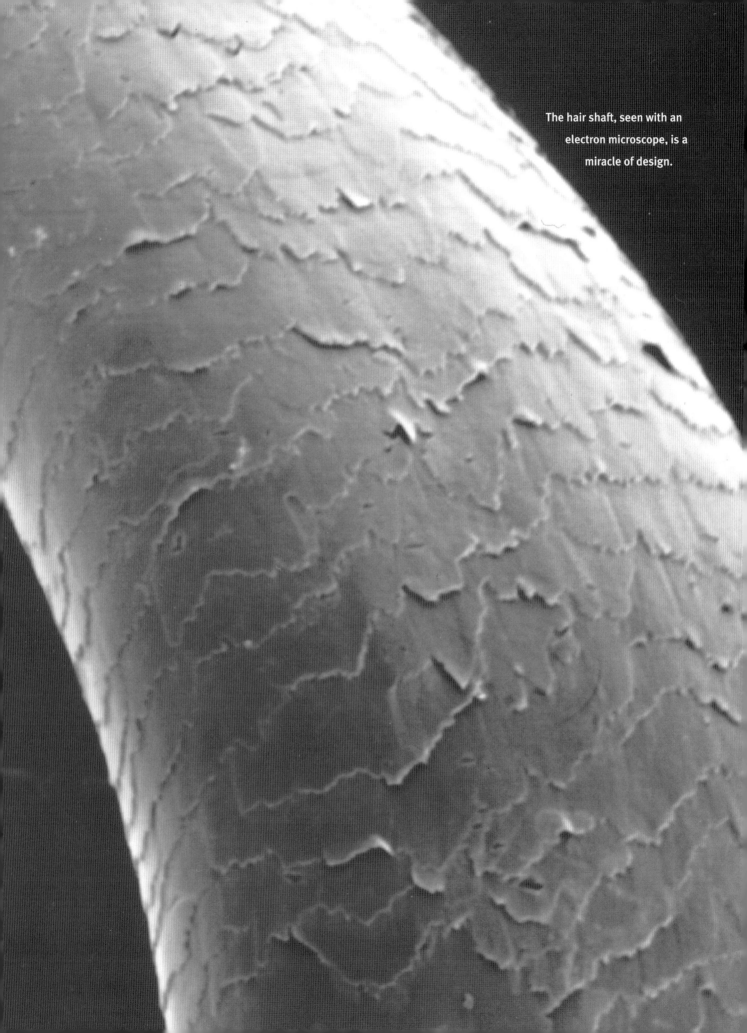

The hair shaft, seen with an electron microscope, is a miracle of design.

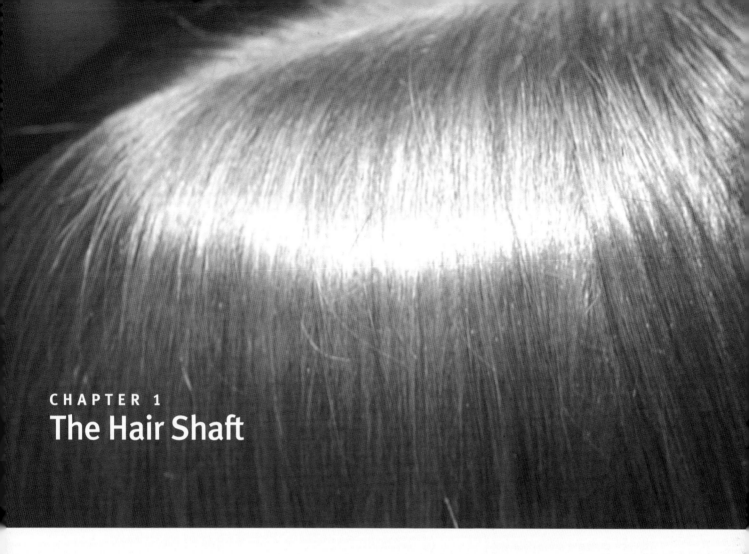

CHAPTER 1
The Hair Shaft

Human beings are all members of just one species of **primate**.
Primates – a group that comprises about 200 species altogether,
including the great apes and the monkeys – form a group of individuals who share certain anatomical characteristics, not all of
which are identical in every individual of the group.

We inherit our particular versions of the features that we share
with other humans from our parents, in whom there is represented the trend of genetic characteristics that has developed over
generations of evolutionary history. We begin our study of the
characteristics of hair with a brief look at the structure of the
hairs themselves.

TYPES OF HAIR

Two types of hair grow on the adult human body:

- **vellus hairs:** these are fine hairs, no more than a centimetre or
  two long, containing little or no pigment and growing from
  hair follicles that have no sebaceous glands

Fabulous shine, with each hair
shaft reflecting light, indicating
truly healthy hair.

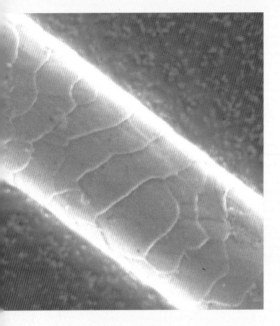

The hair shaft from a newborn child, showing the closely overlapping cells of the cuticle.

The hair shaft of a close relative of ours (though not the closest) – the orang utan. It is almost identical to that of a human hair.

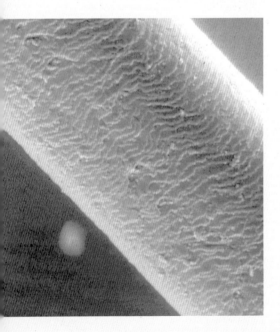

- **terminal hairs:** these are the 'normal' long, thick hairs of the scalp and of the skin, face, chest and arms growing from follicles with sebaceous glands. Hairs in these so-called 'terminal follicles' can gradually become thinner and shorter, eventually looking rather like vellus hairs, in male and female pattern baldness.

The overall appearance of a child's hair, and its appearance in adulthood if it is left to grow unattended, are based on the shape and nature of the 100,000 or so hair shafts on the individual's scalp. In turn, the shape of each of the hair shafts depends, at least in part, on the shape of the hair follicle from which it is derived; it is also probable that the control of formation of the various hair proteins is important. We do not yet precisely know how this mechanism operates, or what its effects may be.

THE HAIR FOLLICLE

The shape of the hair follicle and the rhythms of hair production are determined by the particular collection of genes we have inherited from our parents, which reflects their own inheritance from thousands of generations of their ancestors, and the effects of mate selection and gene sharing among them.

Until the development of modern transport systems travelling was relatively difficult, and groups of people of different customs tended to remain in isolation from each other. These two constraints of geography and culture tended to preserve 'sets' wherein offspring resembled their neighbours: their genes, and hence their hair forms (and skin pigments), would have been similar. These constraints are gradually disappearing from most of the world today.

The follicles on a single head may give rise to a variety of hair shapes representing different so-called 'racial' types (a term that is probably erroneous – see page 25), as well as many abnormal hairs. Within this variety, however, it is the predominant hair shape that determines the overall effect.

THE STRUCTURE OF THE HAIR SHAFT

The hair shaft is essentially a flexible rod of compressed material, a protein known as **keratin**. Keratin is rich in the high-sulphur amino acid cystine, and is a constituent of nails and skin as well as of hair.

A cross-section of a fully mature and keratinised hair shaft reveals the major components of the structure:

- the **cuticle**, which is the outermost layer
- the **cortex**, forming the bulk of the shaft
- the **medulla**, the central core of the hair (not always present).

Cuticle

The cuticle consists of flattened cells arranged along the hair shaft like tiles on a roof, repeated at intervals of approximately every 10 microns. In an untreated (virgin) hair they overlap tightly, minimising the movement of water and other substances in and out of the underlying cortex. The scales of an intact cuticle are smooth and reflect light, and the hair appears glossy and healthy.

It is widely believed that the integrity of the hair shaft cannot be maintained without the cuticle. Recent work suggests that this is not an absolute requirement and that the hair shaft can survive without the cuticle, but not for long periods.

Cortex

The cortex consists of long keratin filaments bound together in a dense matrix containing fats (lipids). These filaments are responsible for the physical and physiological characteristics of the hair shaft, in particular its ability to recover from stretching and flexing.

The protein bundles in the hair shaft are held together by millions of chemical bonds, which are of two major types: **disulphide bonds** and **hydrogen bonds**. The powerful disulphide bonds give hair its great tensile strength, and can only be changed permanently by chemical processes such as perming or relaxing. The weak hydrogen bonds, on the other hand, are easily broken in the presence of water, and rearranged by

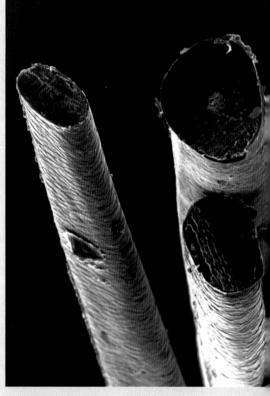

Different shapes of hair shafts, as shown by the electron microscope. All the structural components can be clearly seen: the scales of the cuticle, the densely packed protein-based cortex and (in the large Oriental hair) the presence of a medulla.

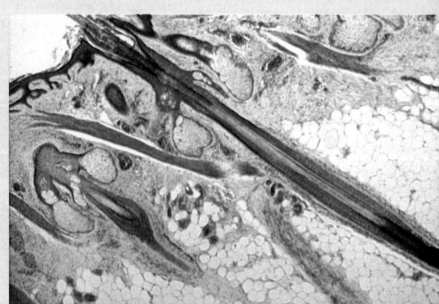

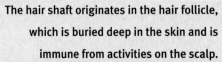

The hair shaft originates in the hair follicle, which is buried deep in the skin and is immune from activities on the scalp.

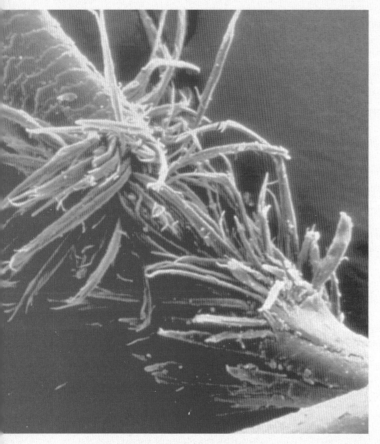

The ultimate effect of severe chemical treatment on hair: rupture of the cortex.

'setting'; these changes are temporary and easily reversed.

The cortex contains granules of pigments (**melanins**). **Eumelanin** (the predominating pigment in the human population) is black-brown, and **phaeomelanin** is reddish-blond. The proportions of these melanin pigments present in the shaft determine the colour of the hair.

Medulla

In humans, a medulla is intermittently found in the pigmented terminal hairs, and is more common in the coarser de-pigmented hairs that develop with ageing. It consists of loosely packed cells and immature protein filaments. It is the least important of the hair's characteristic constituent structures, and is probably a relic of our mammalian ancestors who needed to conserve heat rather more than we do.

THE SCALP HAIR

The hair shaft is technically dead.

The human scalp carries some 100,000–150,000 hair follicles: the number in any individual is determined in the embryo stage and remains unaltered thereafter.

The density of the scalp follicles decreases with age as the scalp area increases, from around 500–700 per cm² at birth to 250–350 per cm² in adulthood.

Each follicle commonly grows a hair continuously for between two and seven years, producing a terminal hair that may grow to as much as a metre in length.

Each follicle on average grows 20 hairs in a lifetime.

Hair follicles in active growth lie in, or just above, the subcutaneous fat of the scalp. Here they are immune from any deleterious effects of materials applied to the scalp. Only severe scarring or systemic factors interfere with hair growth.

Weight for weight, the hair shaft is stronger and more resilient than steel.

The hairs on a human head may have a diversity of shapes, which together determine the overall appearance of the hair and the ability to achieve styling success.

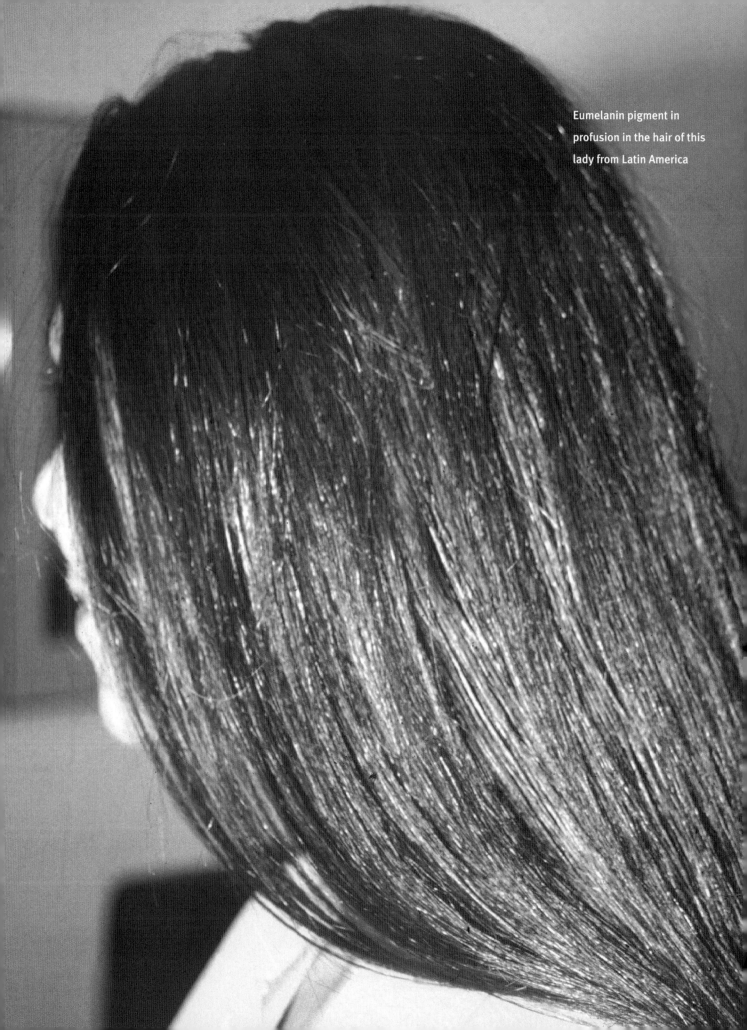

Eumelanin pigment in profusion in the hair of this lady from Latin America

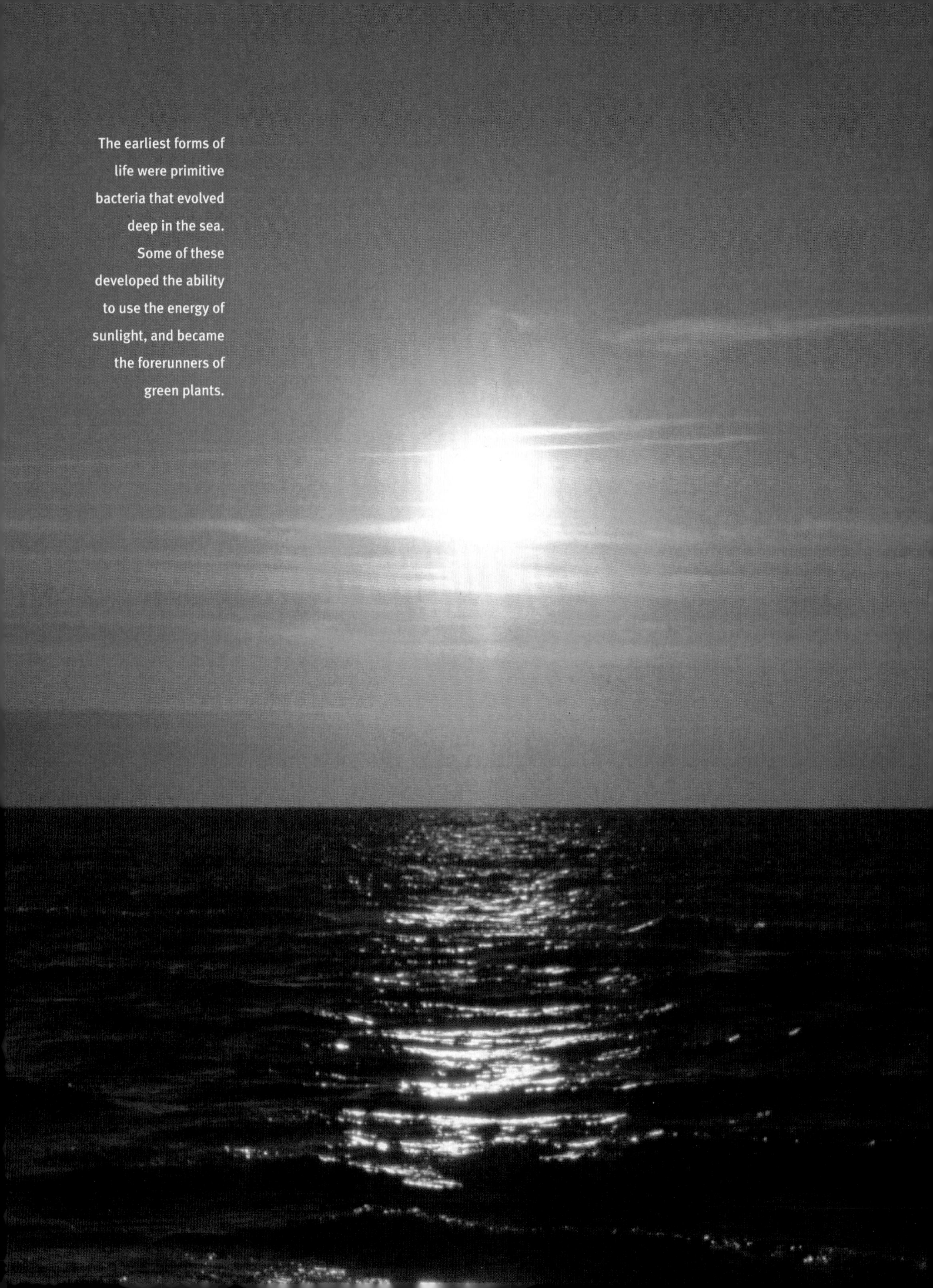

The earliest forms of
life were primitive
bacteria that evolved
deep in the sea.
Some of these
developed the ability
to use the energy of
sunlight, and became
the forerunners of
green plants.

CHAPTER 2
The Human Diaspora

If we are to understand the astonishing diversity of the physical characteristics of humans – including hair forms, among many other features – in the context of our common origins, we need to understand something of the way in which our ancestors spread around the world of their day and how this has affected us today.

The planet Earth is some four billion years old, and for much of that time has carried no living organisms at all upon its surface. the first tiny and primitive living things seem to have appeared perhaps a billion years ago (the evidence is scanty), but for most of the huge tracts of time since then no creature anything like the humans we know appeared on Earth. Yet within the merest blink of an evolutionary eye, the world has been populated first by recognisably human ancestors belonging to species now extinct, and then by modern humans – the species that scientists identify by the name of *Homo sapiens*, meaning (in Latin) 'wise person'.

Many scientists believe that some five million years ago, in what is now East Africa, a new kind of ground-living ape evolved from the tree-dwelling apes of the region. These were our earliest

On this evolutionary timeline, one millimetre corresponds to a period of about 5 million years. This, coincidentally, is the length of time that has passed since the earliest recognisable hominids first saw the light. The lifetime of modern *Homo sapiens* can only be represented on a diagram like this by a line so fine as to be invisible to the naked eye.

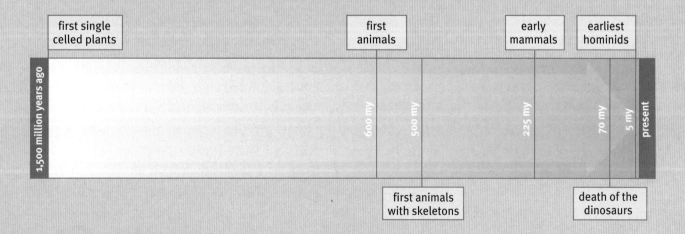

first single celled plants

first animals

early mammals

earliest hominids

1,500 million years ago

600 my

500 my

225 my

70 my

5 my

present

first animals with skeletons

death of the dinosaurs

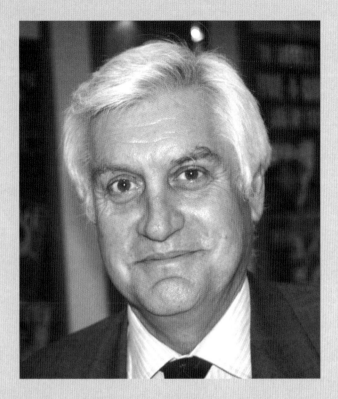

An example of today's *Homo sapiens*, both knowledgeable and wise. We can only guess what the tribal elders of the early human communities looked like, however.

identifiable human ancestors. They began to walk upright regularly, and later on developed tool-making skills, along with an increase in meat-eating. Around perhaps two million years ago, further changes led to the evolution of the first humans, classified as *Homo erectus* ('erect person'). It has been suggested that their ape-like body hair was lost around this time, simultaneously with the development of increased numbers of sweat glands that – then as now – controlled the regulation of their body temperature. Conditions allowed these early peoples to survive and even flourish. (Much of this is necessarily conjecture and there are large gaps in our knowledge.)

Subsequently groups of these individuals spread into Asia and then into Europe, via the Middle East, over hundreds of thousands of years, adapting to the harsher environments they found there, and living as primitive hunter-gatherers. New forms of human, such as the Neanderthals of Europe, evolved. Some 150,000 years ago, within the populations that stayed behind in Africa, *Homo sapiens* evolved, and they too spread out, eventually reaching every part of the world.

Homo sapiens undertook very rapid global migration (see the map on pages 16-17), perhaps interbreeding with existing populations outside of Africa, but eventually these were largely or totally replaced. This hypothesis sees the present 'racial' groups (described in Chapter 3) as being primarily descended from one main population originating in a single region, and later spreading outwards, although why and how the 'racial' differences appeared is not fully understood. As has often been the case with migrating species, older populations were in the main replaced by more successful later arrivals. Most if not all of the earliest populations having now vanished, including the Neanderthals, humankind is seen as genetically almost homogeneous: the physical differences in body height and breadth, and skin and hair colour variations, vividly apparent though they may seem to us, result from only tiny differences in the makeup of our genes.

Biochemical studies of the cells of many different humans have also provided strong evidence supporting the view that modern humans are all descended from a single group that came from one general area – Africa.

While Africa seems to be the source of populations elsewhere in the world, new lineages have arisen in the emergent populations. Other regions of the world have both 'African' and non-African lineages. The populations of Asia, Australia and New Guinea were founded by successively smaller numbers of lineages. This pattern might arise because population 'bottle-necking' had reduced the number of lineages. Some studies suggest that, at various times in the past, this bottlenecking may have been so severe in Europe that most of the present population of the continent derives from just seven distinct clans.

We can calculate that lineages diverge at a rate of about 2-4% per million years. The oldest population group outside Africa with no African features is estimated to be 90,000 to 180,000 years old (though these figures should be treated with caution).

Modern humans appeared in different parts of the world at widely differing times.

The Far East

South-west Asia was first colonised by modern humans at a relatively early date, as much as 100,000 years ago. They did not get a permanent foothold here until much later, however. They may have dispersed along the coasts of southern Asia around 80,000 years ago. The date of their first appearance in China is uncertain, but fossil evidence suggests that it was at least 30,000 years ago.

BERINGIA

Ice free corridor opens c.12–14,000

10,500

Clovis sites
occupied around
11,500–11,000

11–10,000

11,22–10,500

10,000

40

early modern
humans reach
Patagonia
11,000

HUMAN ORIGINS AND HAIR DIVERSITY

- Human evolution appears to have been initiated as the Earth's
  climate started to cool, some 25 million years ago. Lush forests
  in Africa, Europe and Asia provided a habitat for tree-dwelling
  apes including an ancestor of gorillas and other great apes, as
  well as of humans.

- 5 million years ago the forests in Africa began to retreat, and in
  the drier East Africa ground-dwelling hominids first appeared.

- 1.9 million years ago our ancestor *Homo erectus* mastered fire
  and tool-making and slowly migrated out of the African
  homeland through tropical Asia and temperate Europe, but
  without reaching the Americas, Australasia or the Arctic regions.

- Modern *Homo sapiens* appeared as recently as 200,000 to
  135,000 years ago in East Africa.

- We do not know what the hair of the first modern humans was
  like. Modern 'African' hair may have developed independently
  after humans migrated out of Africa. Similar types of hair are
  seen in south-east Asia and Australasia, but we do not know
  whether these also developed independently.

- By 90,000 years ago modern humans had reached the Middle
  East. By 75,000 years ago they had spread into East Asia, and
  by 40,000 years ago into Europe.

- 10,000 years ago all the Earth except Antarctica and parts of the
  Arctic was populated, although total world population may have
  been as few as 3 million persons.

- Small 'sets' of closely related peoples would probably have
  served as the template for hair types in these ancient times.

- We do not yet know how, why or when human hair diversity
  began.

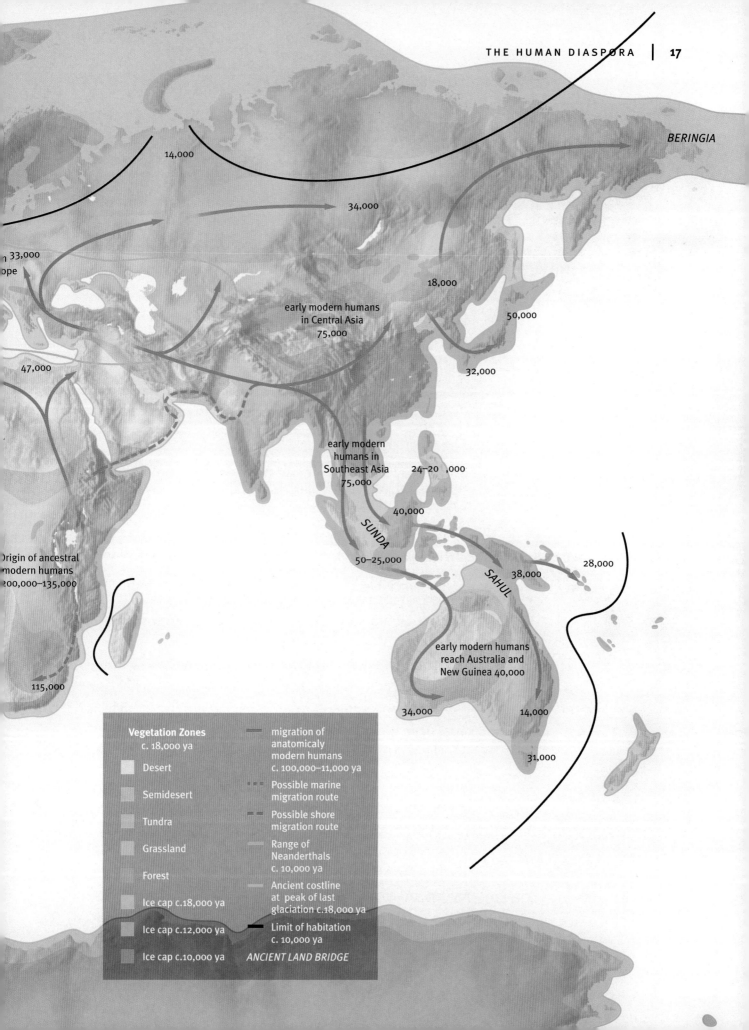

BERINGIA

14,000

34,000

33,000
ope

47,000

early modern humans
in Central Asia
75,000

18,000

50,000

32,000

early modern
humans in
Southeast Asia
75,000

24–20 ,000

40,000

SUNDA

50–25,000

28,000

38,000

SAHUL

Origin of ancestral
modern humans
200,000–135,000

early modern humans
reach Australia and
New Guinea 40,000

34,000

14,000

115,000

31,000

Vegetation Zones
c. 18,000 ya

☐ Desert

☐ Semidesert

☐ Tundra

☐ Grassland

☐ Forest

☐ Ice cap c.18,000 ya

☐ Ice cap c.12,000 ya

☐ Ice cap c.10,000 ya

— migration of
anatomicaly
modern humans
c. 100,000–11,000 ya

---- Possible marine
migration route

---- Possible shore
migration route

— Range of
Neanderthals
c. 10,000 ya

— Ancient costline
at peak of last
glaciation c.18,000 ya

— Limit of habitation
c. 10,000 ya

ANCIENT LAND BRIDGE

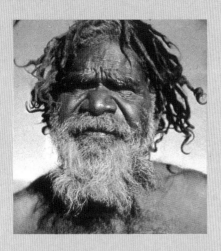

The aboriginal people of Australia and New Guinea can be considered as a distinct group. The skin is dark and the hair is predominantly wavy or frizzy, with blondness in children (lost in adulthood) being common.

Australasia

Although there were considerable expanses of water along the migration route, humans reached Australia at least 60,000 years ago. North Australians are closer to Melanesians than are others, and the Tasmanians (now extinct) also differed slightly from other Australian populations. There was greater variation at many times before 6,000 years ago. The diversity of physical features among early Australians was merely variation on only one fundamentally similar form.

Europe

The earliest *Homo sapiens* may have been excluded from Europe at first by the long-established presence of Neanderthal people, as they appeared there only about 40,000 years ago – a time when Australia had long been colonised.

The Americas

There is currently great debate about the early colonisation of the Americas. Early 'Americans' arrived there relatively recently, from various parts of north-eastern Asia. There may have been a first movement before 20,000 years ago, followed by a second one about 12,000 years ago that was held up until the ice caps formed at the peak of the last Ice Age melted. It may have been this latter group that gave rise to most of the Native Americans. People like the Arctic Inuit probably represent even later migrations from Asia.

There is certainly considerable variation in physical form among the native American populations, which might result from differences among arriving migrant groups. It might also arise from evolution within the groups themselves. All the New World populations, North and South, have characteristics that place them within the Oriental group.

HAIR DIVERSITY AND HUMAN NUMBERS

The differences between the world of today and that of our earliest ancestors are uncountable and almost unimaginable. One of the most marked has been the relatively recent explosive growth in the human population.

The early population movements described above present the sharpest possible contrast to the heaving masses and rapid transportation systems of today. They would have involved tiny close-knit groups of individuals, moving slowly into regions quite unknown to them. Our ancestors depended on hunting, gathering and, more recently, fishing for survival. Food was (and still is in surviving hunter-gathering societies) required not only for subsistence but also for feasting, and played a role in 'mate selection'. The exchange of 'marriage' partners between bands led to the formation of widespread 'mating networks' that linked families over large areas. Towards the end of the Palaeolithic period these may have become more restricted, perhaps because of the pressures of population growth and the emergence of local ethnic identity. Other factors, such as the global rise of sea level that followed the melting of the ice caps about 12,000 years ago, would also have cut populations off from each other. Gene sharing and hair characteristics would have been founded in these close networks. But we do not yet know exactly how or why diversity occurred.

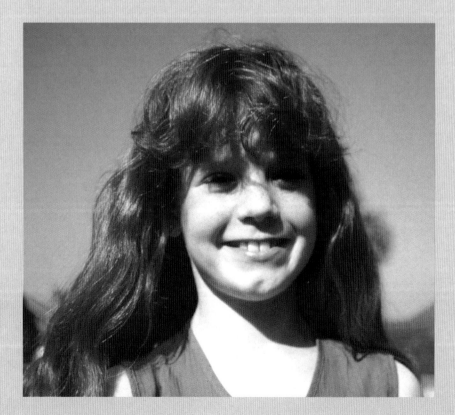

Intense red hair — a characteristic of a European set (Celtic) now concentrated in the extreme west, but seen also in isolated pockets throughout the world.

Estimates of world population size before the advent of wide-spread agriculture some 12,000 to 10,000 years ago generally range from 5 to 10 million people, and the highest figure – calculated on the basis of the largest numbers of hunter-gatherers that the world could support – is only 15 million.

By 1000 A.D. the total world population is estimated to have reached 400 million, with growth steadily accelerating. This led to an astonishing three billion by 1960 – and this number has since doubled in only 40 years!

The early communities were small, and their ranges were bounded by geographical barriers such as mountains, seas and forests. The characteristics of groups would most likely have been concentrated, these concentrations being constrained by numbers which were themselves constrained within geography. Only a few decades ago such genetic concentrations could still be found in villages in the remoter parts of the developed countries, and they still persist throughout most of the Third World.

In the last few thousand years, however, and increasingly in the past five hundred, mass migrations of people over land and sea have resulted in very different societies. Humans have been extremely mobile compared with other species, as demonstrated by their spread over the Earth in the past ten millennia. Within the past few centuries, millions of Europeans and Africans migrated, willingly or otherwise, to both North and South America, Europeans to Australasia and South Africa, and Oriental people south to other parts of Asia and to the Americas (see the map on pages 22-23). The early populations of south-east China increased dramatically in numbers after the last Ice Age (about 10,000 years ago), and have been highly influential in subsequent migrations southward in that region. Their hair characteristics can even be seen in certain European populations, subtly combined with others, suggesting a 'drift of genes'.

The tightly curled dark hair indicates genes from sub-Saharan Africa, but Indo-European genes are present too.

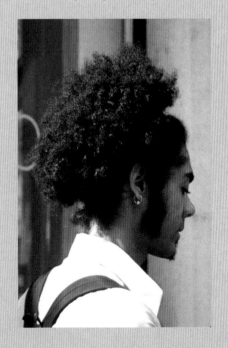

Today individuals can travel from one side of the world to another in a few hours – and many of them do. The original local 'stock', usually with very distinct regional or district characteristics, is now being forged into increasing diversity. Only in a few very large countries such as China and India are the movements of sets limited that pronounced hair characteristics are still maintained with any degree of uniformity.

GENE FLOW

Variety can only exist in populations, not in individuals, but exactly what constitutes a population may be difficult to define. A population may share space and genes, but usually only an isolated community will form a population from a geneticist's point of view. For most of the evolutionary history of *Homo sapiens* populations have been small sets of this kind, existing in isolation for long periods during which the group continues to evolve slowly. From time to time, however, these groups were disrupted by population expansion, migration, invasion and intermixture. Thus periods of differentiation in small populations have been interrupted by periods of gene flow.

Dramatic increases in mobility over the past few centuries have accelerated this process, and broadened mating circles all over the world. In many societies, discrete units have all but vanished: for example, despite previous restrictions there are now large mixed groups in South Africa, the USA, South America and Polynesia, especially Hawaii. In other communities, however, especially those isolated by geography or religion, the process has only just begun.

Gene flow into a population brings new characteristics to the group and increases its diversity. On the other hand, gene flow between populations – the exchange of genes between the groups – tends to make the populations more similar. If gene flow occurs in both directions it can eventually make the populations genetically identical. Gene flow, in short, is the great homogenising *and* the great diversifying factor in human evolution.

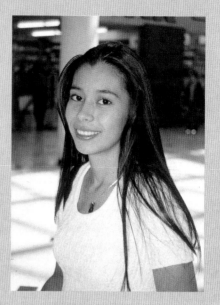

Oriental and Indo-European genes in the New World: a majestic head of hair

Indo-European genes meet with African genes, here giving a preponderance of light-coloured curls.

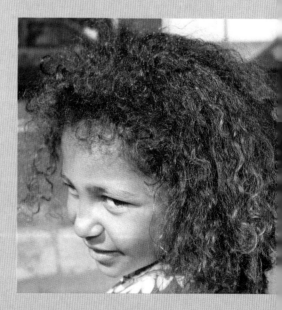

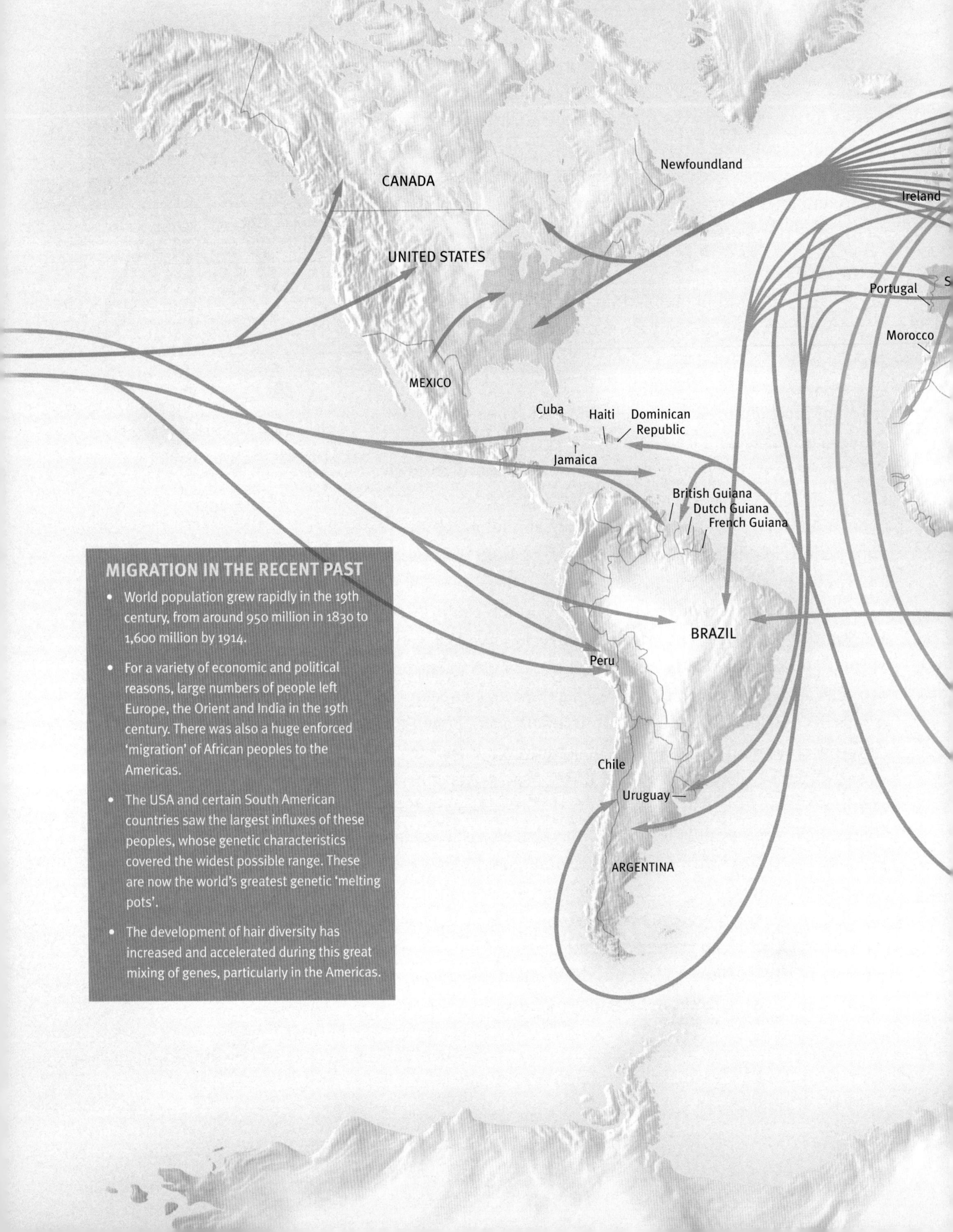

GREENLAND

Newfoundland

CANADA

UNITED STATES

MEXICO

Ireland

Portugal

Morocco

Cuba   Haiti   Dominican
                 Republic

Jamaica

British Guiana
Dutch Guiana
French Guiana

BRAZIL

Peru

Chile

Uruguay

ARGENTINA

MIGRATION IN THE RECENT PAST

- World population grew rapidly in the 19th century, from around 950 million in 1830 to 1,600 million by 1914.

- For a variety of economic and political reasons, large numbers of people left Europe, the Orient and India in the 19th century. There was also a huge enforced 'migration' of African peoples to the Americas.

- The USA and certain South American countries saw the largest influxes of these peoples, whose genetic characteristics covered the widest possible range. These are now the world's greatest genetic 'melting pots'.

- The development of hair diversity has increased and accelerated during this great mixing of genes, particularly in the Americas.

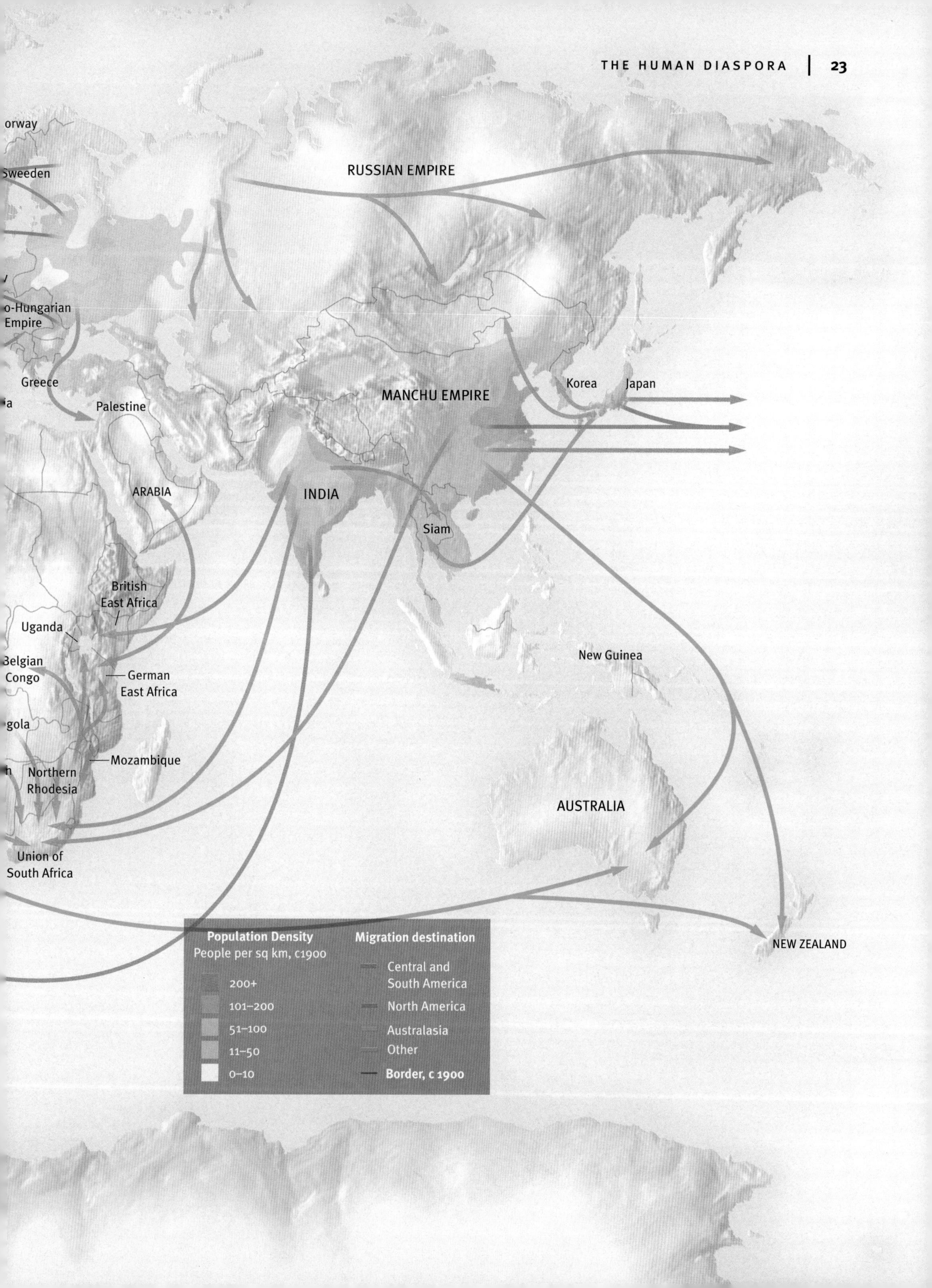

orway

Sweeden

o-Hungarian
Empire

Greece

a

RUSSIAN EMPIRE

MANCHU EMPIRE

Korea   Japan

Palestine

ARABIA

INDIA

Siam

British
East Africa

Uganda

Belgian
Congo

German
East Africa

New Guinea

gola

Northern
Rhodesia

Mozambique

AUSTRALIA

Union of
South Africa

NEW ZEALAND

Population Density
People per sq km, c1900

200+

101–200

51–100

11–50

0–10

Migration destination

Central and
South America

North America

Australasia

Other

Border, c 1900

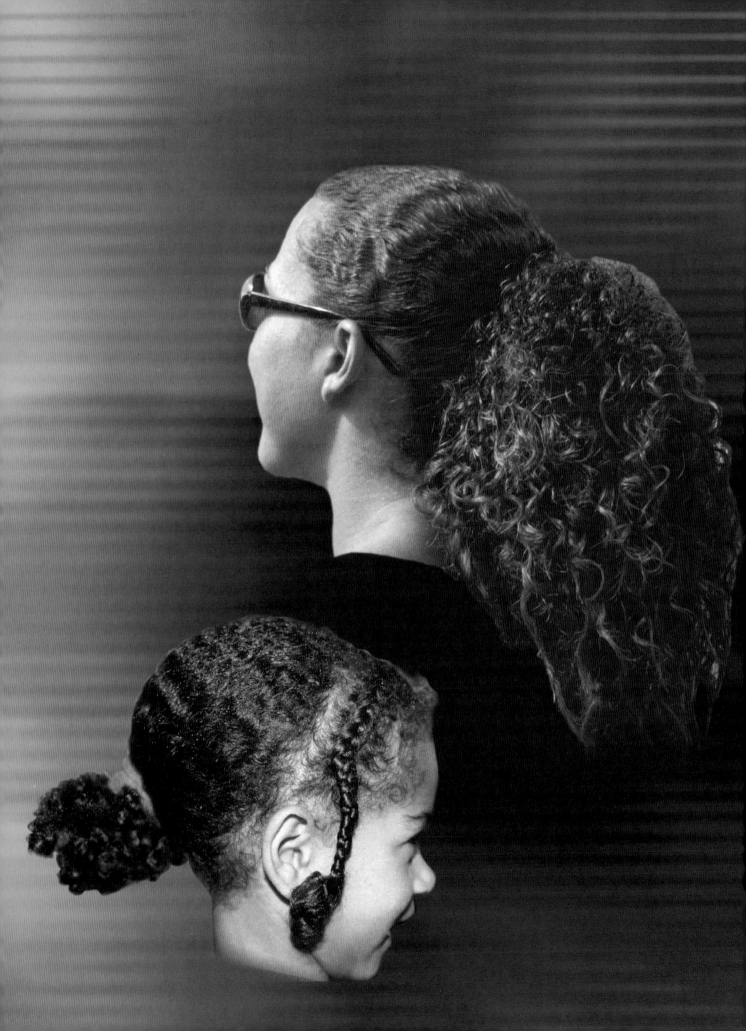

CHAPTER 3
'Ethnic' Hair Today

Historically the word 'ethnic' has been employed to describe certain physical characteristics of large groups or 'sets' of peoples, and has been adapted as a media or marketing concept. It was used to convey not only differences in physical characteristics but also more loosely, and perhaps more appropriately, the presence or practice of certain traditions.

Traditionally hair shaft differences have been described in terms of category labels such as 'Caucasoid', 'Mongoloid' and 'Negroid'. This classical but inflexible approach seems to indicate that if one comes from a certain region one's hair is inevitably of a certain type. But this was never true. We do not know why hair grows with such different characteristics, and until geneticists have identified all the products of the genes in the human chromosomes, and the functions of those products, we cannot hope to understand the details of the processes involved.

Nor do we yet have an agreed nomenclature. In this publication we have used some of the traditional geographical terms such as 'Oriental' or 'Indo-European' or 'African'. We should remember, however, that these terms are simplifications, since some genetic studies suggest that Africa has as much variation as the rest of the world put together! The varieties of hair seen in the Americas, where today's larger population groups have lived for only about 300 years and there has been tremendous gene flow between groups, are almost impossible to describe. And there are many other peoples, each with their own distinctive mix of characteristics, who do not fit into any of the major geographical groupings – people such as the Ainu of Japan, the Andamanese Islanders and the Bushmen of southern Africa. There are also populations in regions like south-east Asia and Melanesia who superficially look 'African', and have an 'African' hair type. It is not yet known whether their hair characteristics come from possessing the same genes for hair type that Africans have, or whether they have developed these characteristics independently.

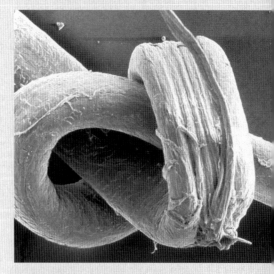

African hair readily forms tight knots, which are impossible to unravel.

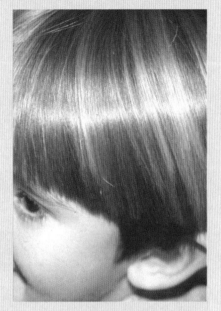

Natural highlights due to differing melanin pigments in a child of Indo-European extraction

INDO-EUROPEAN ('CAUCASIAN') HAIR

The traditional use of the term 'Caucasian' was based on old assumptions about origins, and where the most perfect examples could be found. In reality there is evidence that these people were already widespread in Europe and western Asia over 10,000 years ago, and it is unclear where they first originated. Successive waves of westward migration over many centuries ensured a constant gene flow, in conjunction with the spread of farming, and perhaps with language spread. It probably happened within groups of similar-looking peoples, and among their descendants hair characteristics vary enormously, from fine, straight blond hair to dense dark curls. Their hair contains mixtures of melanin pigments: the reddish-brown phaeomelanin is common in north-west Europe and especially among the descendants of the Celtic peoples, while in southern parts of the Indo-European region eumelanin is the predominant pigment.

Among this group the hair shaft shows tremendous variability. It generally has a slightly flattened or oval cross-section. 'Straight' hair is characterised by a certain diameter range (50-90 microns)

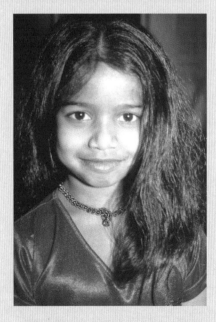

The people of the Indian subcontinent and their descendants represent the southernmost element of the Indo-Europeans who probably migrated out of the eastern Caucasus thousands of years ago

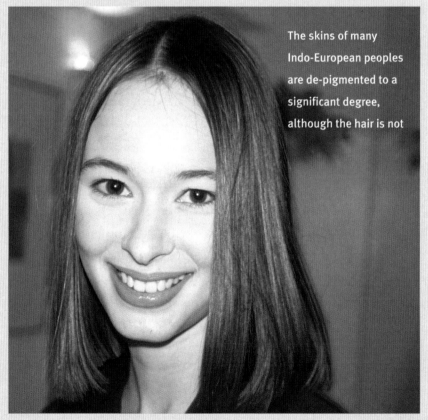

The skins of many Indo-European peoples are de-pigmented to a significant degree, although the hair is not

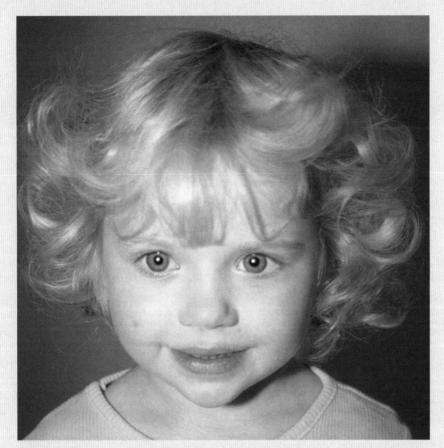

The natural curls of childhood, here pigmented with phaeomelanin, may be due to the expression of particular keratins in the hair follicles as well as to the hair shape

A child of the southern Mediterranean. People from this region show a wide range of hair characteristics

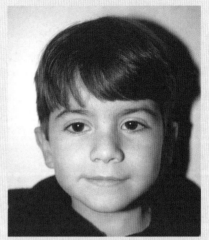

and a relatively untwisted structure. Curly hair is much more highly twisted. It is not known where, why and when this diversity arose, but the open geography of the Indo-European area presumably allowed easier migration and greater mixing with genes originating from the Middle East and northern Africa.

Very fine hair (diameter less than 50 microns) tends to be most frequently seen in Scandinavia and areas where there has been gene sharing with Scandinavian peoples, such as north-western Europe and the UK. This characteristic curiously persisted from the early farming communities and then in the Vikings and their descendants. In the 19th and 20th centuries it was carried into North American, Australasian and southern African populations.

In southern parts of Europe hair tends to contain more eumelanin, and from north to south down the long 'boot' of Italy there is an apparent gradation of hair colour from light to dark. The Indian subcontinent shows a further enhancement of this gene cline from the original Indo-Europeans, but the causes of the heavier pigmentation of southern Indian peoples are unknown.

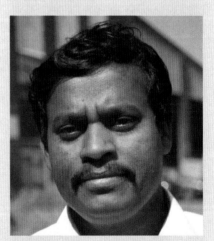

Eumelanin predominates in the hair and skin of peoples of the Indian subcontinent. Dark pigments are more associated with heat conservation in the skin than protection against UV radiation. There is no known advantage in dark hair colour.

'ORIENTAL' HAIR

Characteristically thick hair – up to 120 microns in diameter – round in shape and with relatively few twists per unit length is seen most often in peoples of the Far Eastern countries (China, Japan and Korea).

In eastern Asia the sets most often seen are characterised by lighter skins that bear pigments giving a yellowish appearance but still have the ability to tan, in association with dark, straight and thick hair in which the predominant pigment is the black-brown eumelanin. The hair forms that have been evident in this population for generations derive directly from the particular characteristics of this hair. The ancestors of these people may have migrated from China and shared their genes with populations to the east and south of their original homelands.

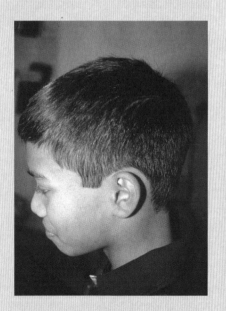

Sri Lanka, whence this boy's family originated, is the region where Indo-Europe and the Orient meet.

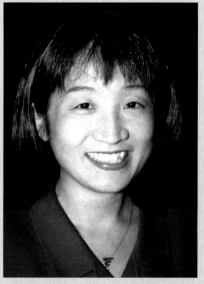

Modern Japanese woman!

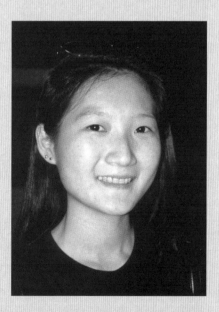

Chinese peoples are strongly linked genetically with most (though not all) other peoples with Oriental characteristics in South-East Asia and North and South America

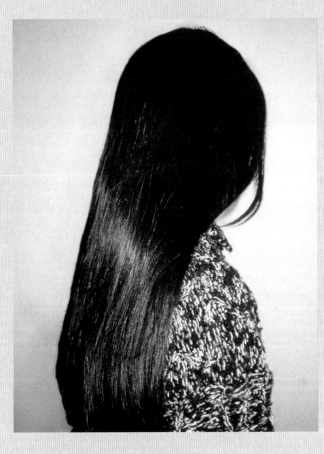

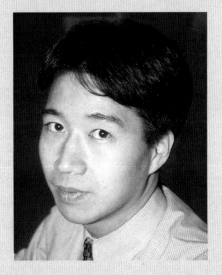

Finer hair is also seen in southern parts of China.

Powerful Oriental hair, with hair shaft diameter up to 120 microns, is common in northern China and Korea.

Finer hair from the Orient can be worn in longer styles; this lady comes from Malaysia.

The intense whorl of Oriental hair; thick cylindrical hair shafts give this hair its characteristically powerful nature – it is often difficult to style if worn short.

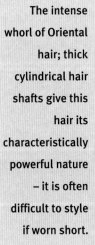

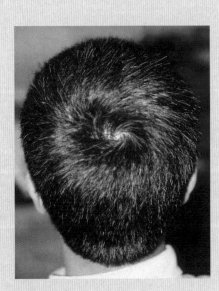

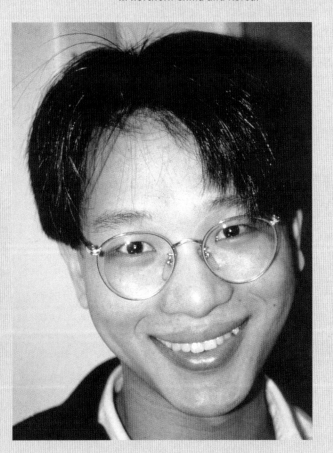

'AFRICAN' (SUB-SAHARAN) HAIR

Hair shafts from peoples whose recent ancestors originated in sub-Saharan Africa, who now live in many countries outside the African continent, tend to have a highly characteristic shape. Hairs are considerably flattened and often grooved, and frequently vary in diameter along a single strand. They tend to be highly twisted, with random reversals in twist direction. The hair is quite sharply kinked at the edges, and is especially vulnerable to damage at such points. This kind of hair tends to be more easily harmed by cosmetic maltreatment than is cylindrical hair, and grooming it requires more force especially when it is dry (see page 46). It is normally densely pigmented with eumelanin. The hair of people from eastern Africa tends to show much less curl, and the origins of its characteristics are not known.

Nor do we know why this 'African' type of hair shaft should be so different from hair seen in most other parts of the world. Given that *Homo sapiens* probably evolved in sub-Saharan Africa during the last 150,000 years, we might suppose that this is the original early hair form and that cylindrical hair evolved later. But all modern populations have changed since then, and the time scale also makes this less likely. Some scientists believe that early humans may have had cylindrical hair, but why, when or how 'African' hair evolved is unknown.

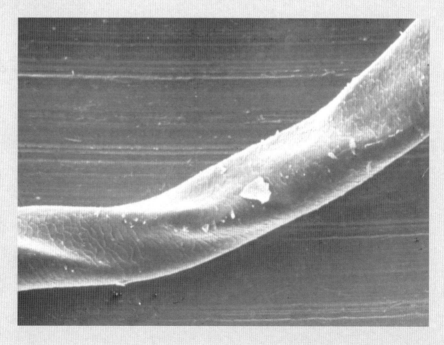

The naturally twisted hair characteristic of peoples of sub-Saharan Africa.

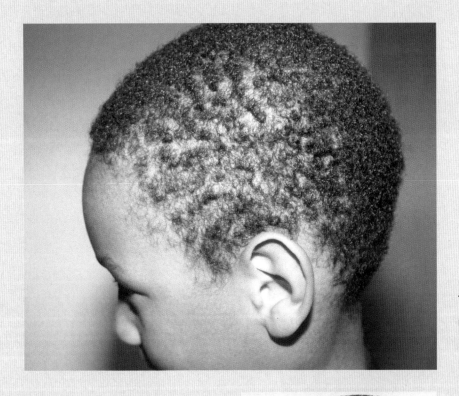

The tight curls of Africa are easy to manage when worn short. Grooming becomes difficult when they are worn longer.

A tight top-knot in African hair; this is a popular style for children, but it can lead to chronic traction damage.

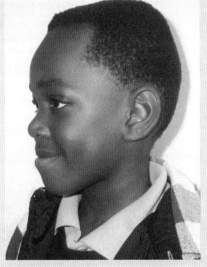

This lady relaxes her hair and then gently reperms it.

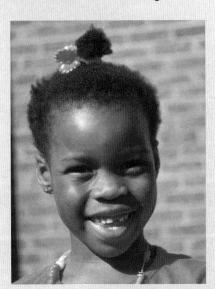

Gene lines for some peoples in southern Africa have been traced back over 120,000 years.

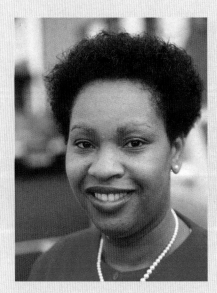

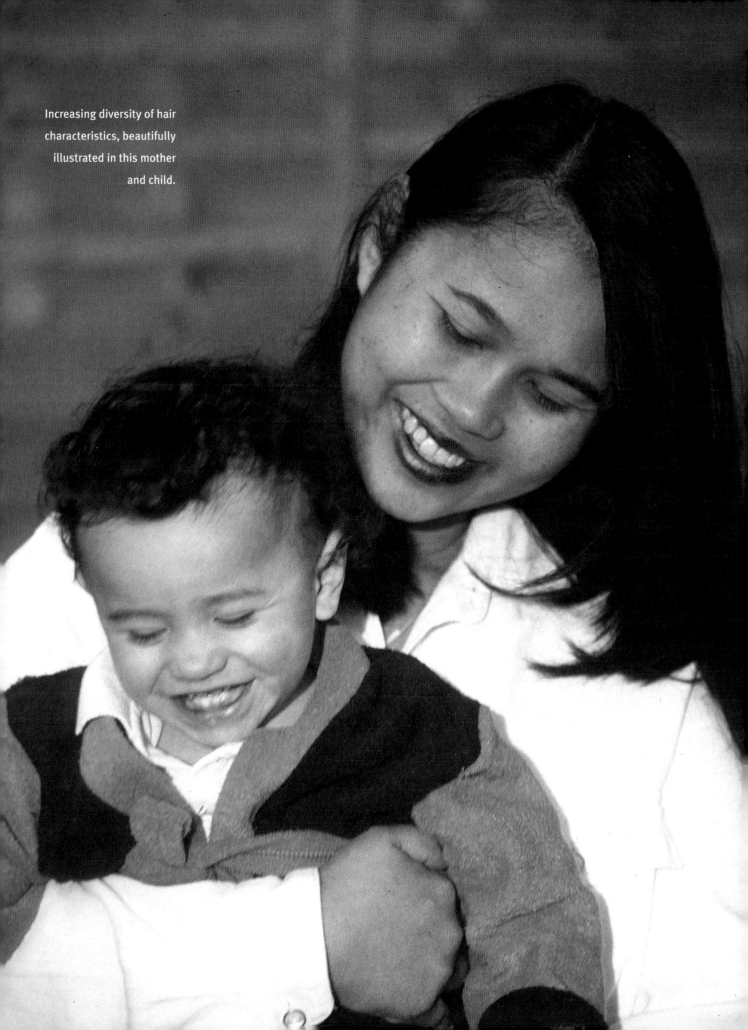

Increasing diversity of hair characteristics, beautifully illustrated in this mother and child.

CHAPTER 4
Hair Characteristics

The function and appearance of one's hair depend on three major characteristics of the hair shaft: its porosity, its elasticity and its texture. These are all to some extent dependent on the predominating shape and structure of the individual hairs. In this chapter we shall look at the enormous range of heritable characteristics of our hair. These characteristics deserve some discussion as they have a significant impact on the way in which hair responds to physical and chemical treatments. They also dictate the aesthetic potential, which we will discuss in Chapter 5.

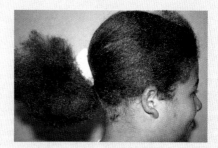

Hair such as this tends to be naturally more porous than straight hair.

POROSITY

The **porosity** of the hair is a measure of its ability to allow moisture to pass through the cuticle into the cortex. In a healthy, undamaged hair shaft, only a minimal amount of water or other substances can penetrate through the cuticle into the cortex.

Weathering after repeated perming and bleaching leads to dry and porous hair. Intensive conditioning may help.

The chemical reactions of perming or hair colouring take place in the cortex. They can only happen if the scales of the cuticle have been separated to some extent to allow the chemicals to penetrate the hair. This is achieved by increasing the temperature or by changing the pH of the environment around the shaft. When the processing of hair is finished, these cuticular scales gradually close again. If the hair is processed too many times the cuticle cannot quite return to its original tightness and the barrier becomes imperfect; as a result the hair can become more porous.

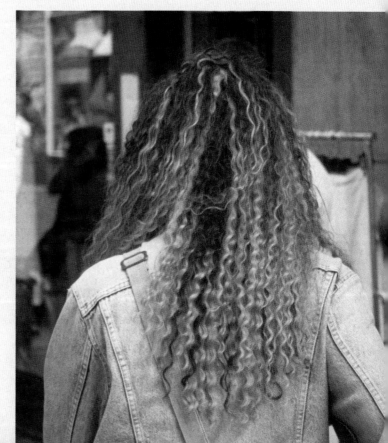

A split end – the final breakdown of the hair shaft after repeated abuse. It cannot be permanently repaired, although modern hair care products may temporarily improve its appearance.

Not only chemical processing, but also overheating from repeated close blow-drying or from curling irons, wind and sunlight can increase the porosity of the hair shaft. If the cuticle becomes significantly damaged, the shaft may become temporarily engorged with water whenever the hair is washed. Immediately after perming the porosity is at a maximum, and the volume of water that can enter the hair shaft may then increase by up to 200 times!

Highly porous hair tends to be dry and eventually fragile, and often contains split ends. Severely damaged hair may fracture and the results may be seen as hair 'loss'. The management of porous hair is currently a prime objective of hair cosmetology and science. Technology to improve the water-retaining potential of the hair shaft is actively being explored at the time of writing.

ELASTICITY AND STRENGTH

Another major characteristic of the hair shaft is its **elasticity**.

Elasticity is a measure of how far the hair can be stretched without losing the ability to spring back to its original length: healthy hair can stretch by about one-third of its length without damage. Hair with poor elasticity will have little or no curl, will tend to break more easily when groomed, and will be less likely to withstand routine chemical treatments such as permanent waving.

The **tensile strength** of hair is related to its elasticity, and is assessed by finding the maximum mass it can support. A single dry hair can support a 100-g weight without breaking. The tensile strength is dependent upon a healthy cortex, which in turn depends largely upon protection by a healthy cuticle.

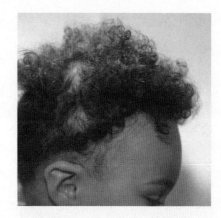

African hair: such tightly curled hair tends to be dry.

TEXTURE

The third major characteristic of hair is its **texture**. Texture is dependent on two factors: the diameter of the individual hair fibre – that is, whether it is coarse or fine – and the feel of the hair, whether harsh, soft, or wiry.

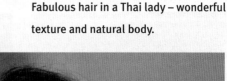

Fabulous hair in a Thai lady – wonderful texture and natural body.

PERMEABILITY

These three major characteristics of the hair shaft – porosity, elasticity and texture – all affect the overall permeability of hair to chemical treatments. When the processing time is judged, both porosity and texture must be taken into account. For example, fine hair will become saturated with waving lotion more quickly than coarser hair, if their porosity is the same. Coarse hair that is very porous, however, will process more quickly than fine hair that is not porous.

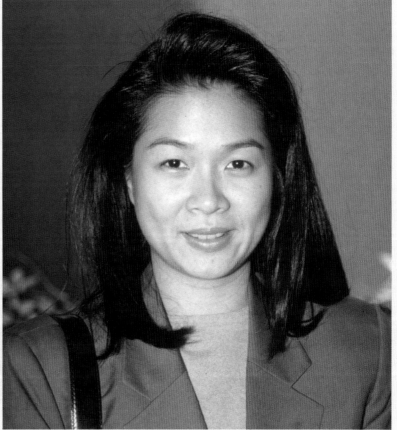

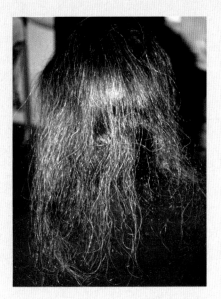

'Ageing' hair.

'Ageing' hair

The characteristics of hair can change over the lifetime of the owner. As we grow older, our ability to grow our hair long declines naturally, and its moisture content tends to diminish. The often-repeated act of washing the hair may also gradually remove some of its component amino acids, further impairing the ability of the cortex to function. Modern hair care products can help to restore this reduction by replacing lost amino acids.

HAIR SHAFT SHAPE AND THE APPEARANCE OF THE HAIR

The shape and the diameter of the hair shaft together largely determine the overall appearance of the hair. Hair with a wide diameter, a nearly circular cross-section and a low twist frequency is more likely to stand erect. The flatter and more ribbon-like the hair, and the higher its twist frequency, the more likely it is to be tightly curled.

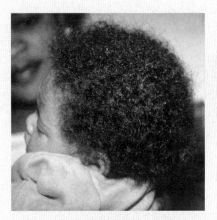

Classical African hair showing intensely dark pigments and tight curls

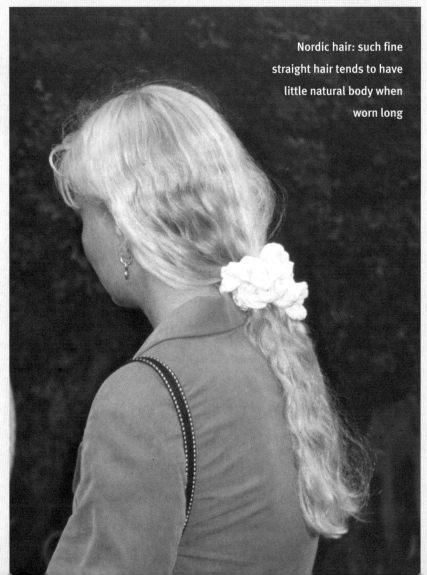

Nordic hair: such fine straight hair tends to have little natural body when worn long

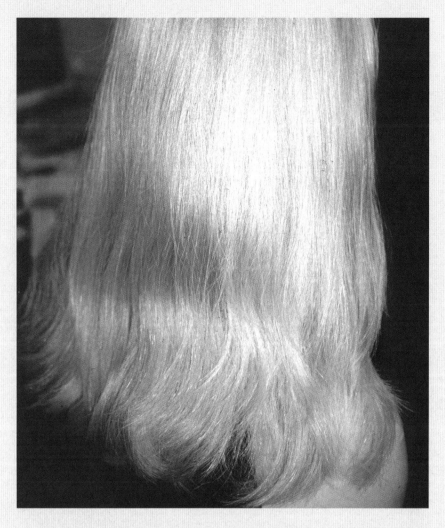

Indo-European peoples show the greatest variety of hair form. This is a typical example of naturally healthy Indo-European hair, even though the tips will have been growing for several years.

The range of hair shapes on an individual's head, together with the hair density, largely determines the overall appearance of the hair and what can be achieved in styling terms. Fine, low-density hair if worn long will tend to be straight and limp (or even lank, if it is oily), and without the use of styling products and blow drying will not hold a style well. High-density hair shafts of moderate to large diameter, with or without natural curl characteristics, will look singularly different, and may be difficult to flatten or shape. Mixtures of hairs of dissimilar shapes result in intermediate hair forms. The result is that a huge range of hair characteristics is found among the world's population today, varying from black and very curly through thick, dark and straight, to pale and fine. In early human populations this diversity was probably much less (see Chapter 2).

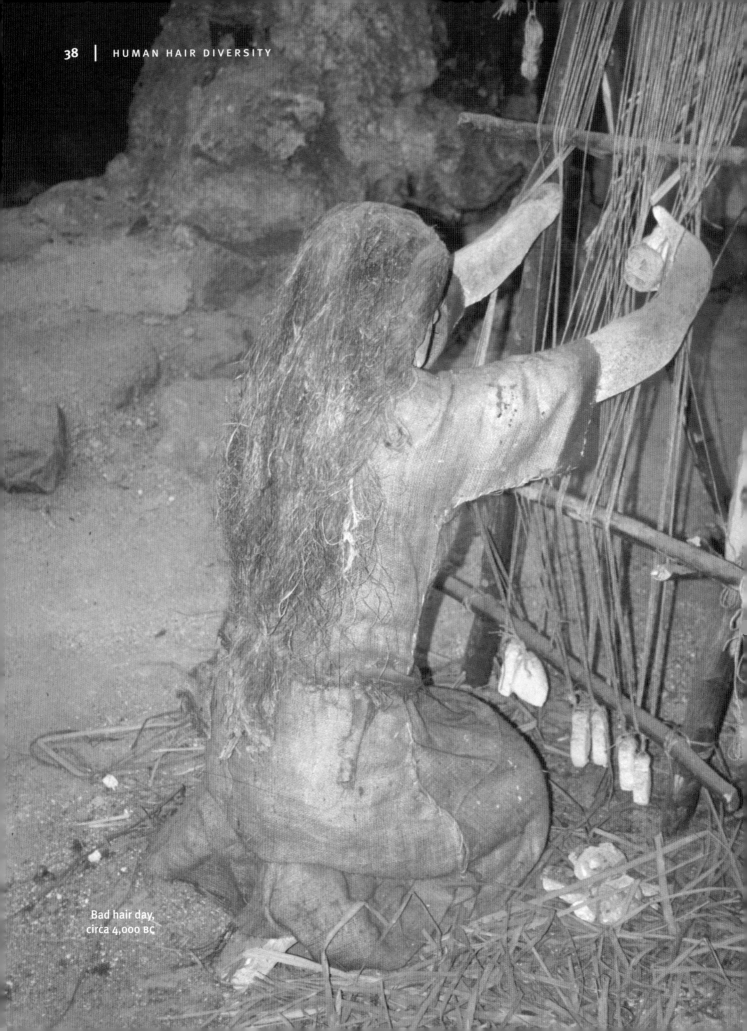

Bad hair day,
circa 4,000 BC

CHAPTER 5
Hair Diversity:
the Art of the Possible

THE IMPORTANCE OF VOLUME

Among the most important aspects of our hair is the appearance of 'volume'. In some people its lack may be due to the onset of male or female pattern baldness. Others find that volume is apparently lessened with the passage of time, or after serious illness, hormonal changes or severe dietary deficiencies. On the other hand people with too much volume, often those with strong Oriental hair, may look to keep this under control. Overly curly hair may also be a problem to manage. Whatever our hair may be like, at some stage in our lives we may well have 'a problem' with it.

We now look at different hair forms.

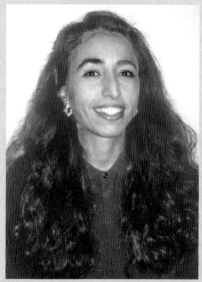

Natural volume.

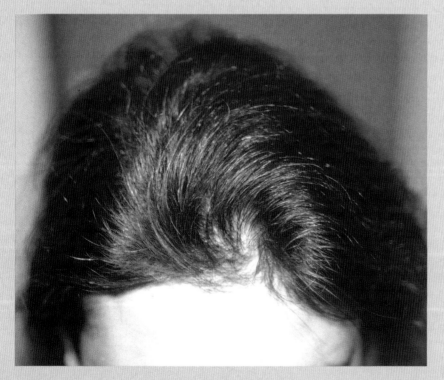

Volume in a lady with
gradual hair loss.

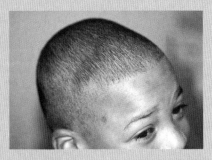

In early childhood even 'African' hair can grow without curl.

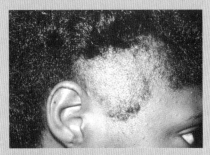

The results of long-term traction on hair at the side of the head.

'AFRICAN' HAIR

As we saw earlier, the hair shaft of modern peoples originating from sub-Saharan Africa is very different from other types of hair. Its shape is distinctive (see page 30), and it tends to be dry: its moisture content may be 5% less than that of Indo-European hair. Partly because of its shape, it is very prone to damage by 'weathering' or by either physical or chemical treatments, particularly when worn long. African hair is only about 85% as strong under tension as Indo-European hair, and is more fragile in both wet and dry conditions. As a result, it is more liable to breakage, especially when mistreated. Considerable force has to be used in combing it (see page 46), and this may give rise to negative electrostatic charges on the hair that contribute to even greater difficulties of management.

Tight braids or ponytails in children, or indeed in adults, may set up a continuous, prolonged tension on the hair follicles. This may result in inflammation in the follicles (**traction folliculitis**) and ultimately to hair loss (**traction alopecia**). If the traction is continued over a period of perhaps three to five years, a permanent scarring alopecia may develop. Where children are concerned, this may appear by early adolescence.

Traction alopecia can be prevented by a change in culture and understanding, and the education of parents and child carers to avoid tightly pulled styles when grooming children's hair.

'African' hair can present a unique and glorious array. It is undeniably more difficult to groom, wash and style than straight hair, but the problems are not insuperable. Many women with this type of hair regularly have it straightened. Unfortunately the tightly curled hair shaft can only be permanently straightened by the reversal of the perming process used to curl straight hair (**relaxing**, see page 59). This makes the hair more manageable, but it does subsequently require substantial additional care because of the damage done by the processing. Relaxed hair can be gently re-permed to induce light curls.

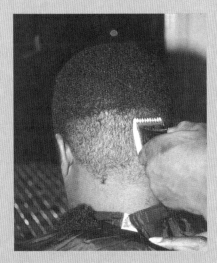

The popular 'fade' cut.

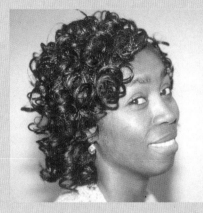

Relaxed and curled hair with extensions, and with sheen imparted by a gel.

Braiding is a popular way to manage 'African' hair in both children and adults. Cosmetic products are designed for this, as all types of hair.

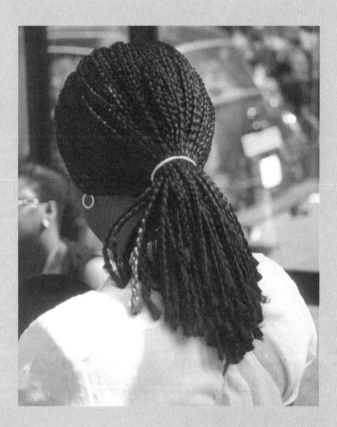

Individuals with African-type hair, both men and women, may manage it by employing an assortment of means, chosen either from a fashion standpoint or for cultural or management reasons.

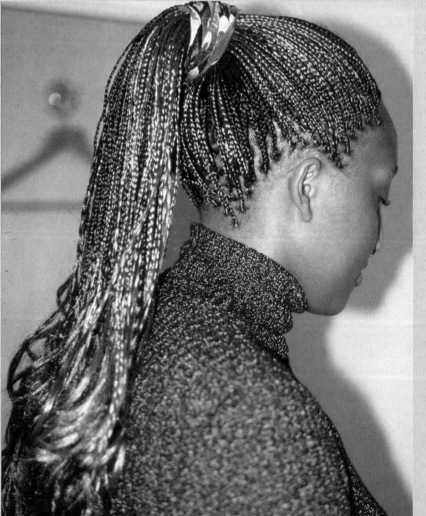

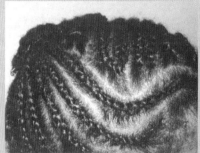

The classical 'cornrow' braiding.

Artificial braids are a way of producing long 'African' hair without the grooming problems. They are often attached to natural braids.

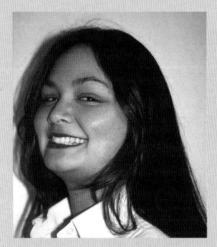

A combination of Indo-European and Oriental characteristics have produced smooth flowing hair in this Anglo-Malayan woman.

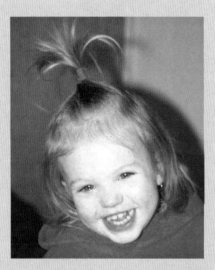

There is a worldwide tendency to create 'cute' styles, especially for 'African' and Indo-European children. Such a style carries a risk of hair breakage, particularly in fine hair.

INDO-EUROPEAN HAIR

There is an immense range of hair forms and colours throughout this huge group of peoples. Many of these characteristics have been carried into the New World. Everything from the fine light straight hair common in the north and west of the region, through red and brown shades and wavy and curly textures, to the thick dark hair seen everywhere in the south and east – all are possible from the genes present. The range of aesthetic possibilities is also immense.

Fine, straight hair can be made more manageable if it is altered to create more volume. This can be done chemically (perming) or by the use of conditioners, volumisers and hair sprays – all products that leave a temporary deposit on the hair. This helps to 'separate' each hair (or, more probably, each group of hairs) from each other. There is potential for 'over-conditioning' of the hair, however, particularly hair that has been chemically abused.

Some individuals try to increase the volume of their hair by setting or perming. Setting straight hair can give waves or curls by temporarily changing the positions of the weak hydrogen bonds in the hair shaft by wetting, rearranging and holding with spray. A permanent wave has its effect by altering the chemistry of the strong disulphide bonds in the hair protein. Very fine Indo-European hair may be hard to perm, however. The reason lies in its structure: the cortex is the part of the hair fibre that holds a perm, and in fine hair the cortex forms a lower proportion of the fibre than cylindrical hair.

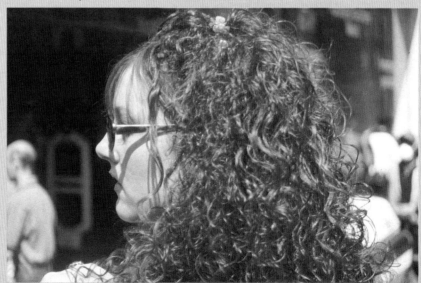

Perming has given character to lank Indo-European hair.

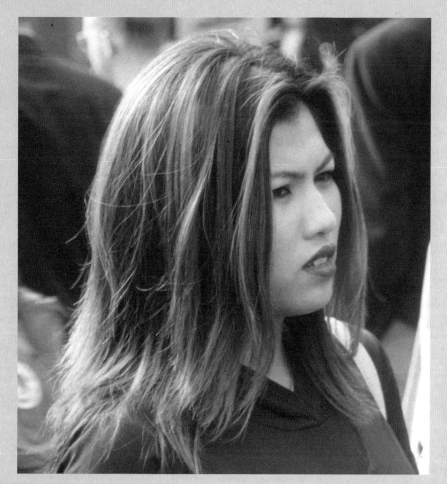

Excessive lightening of Oriental hair not only can create a startling effect but also causes serious weathering.

Beautifully glossy, healthy Oriental hair.

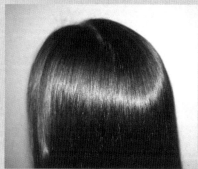

'ORIENTAL' HAIR

The robust straight hair shaft commonly seen in the Far East may be very difficult to style, particularly if worn short. It may become spiky, especially if washed in harsh surfactants. It is difficult to perm, and requires additional concentrations of perming solution. The reason is the stout, cylindrical nature of these hair shafts: unlike the more flattened hair of other groups, they do not flex readily in any particular preferred direction. Perm failures are not uncommon.

Oriental hair is usually black or shades of brown. Changing the colour of this hair—heavily pigmented with eumelanin—is difficult and results most usually in brown or even red highlights. Attempts to cover grey hairs can result in strange tints, and it is only practicable to change the colour from lighter to darker. Bleaching destroys the eumelanin, and tends to produce red-tinged hair as well as leading to increased weathering.

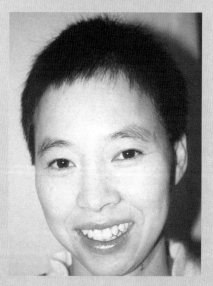

Short Oriental hair may be difficult to manage. The robust cylindrical hairs produce a spiky style, which might be helped by cosmetic products.

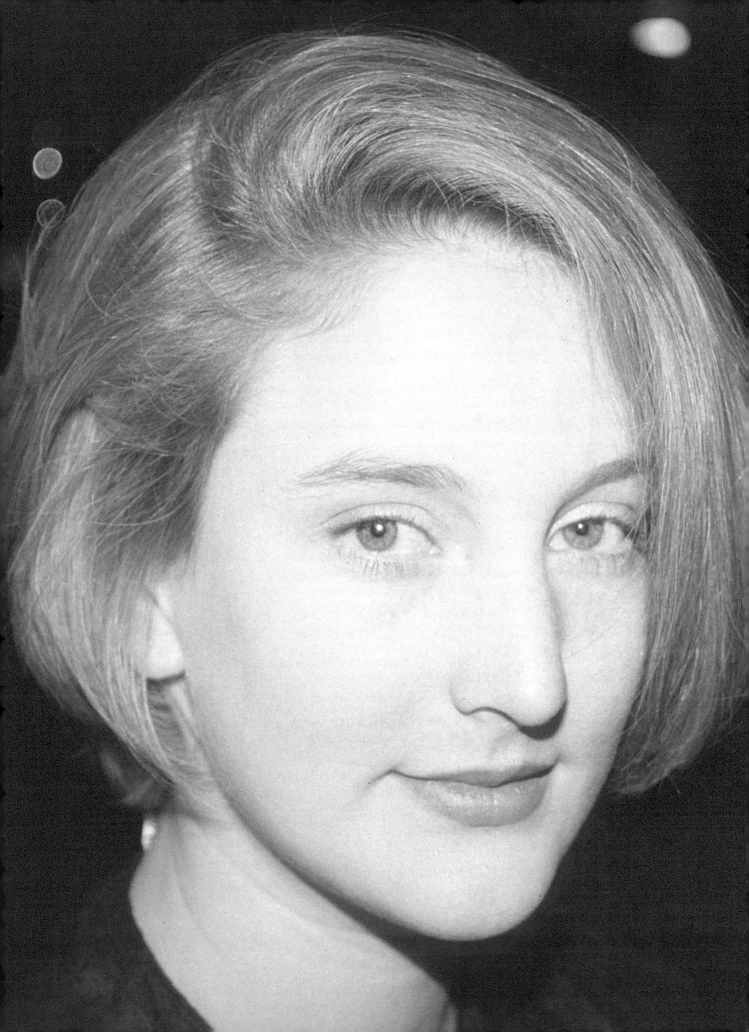

CHAPTER 6

Hair Diversity and Everyday Hair Care

Our hair is an essential part of the totality of our genetic inheritance, and there is nothing whatever we can do on a cosmetic basis that will permanently alter its basic characteristics while it is in the hair follicle. Nevertheless, the cosmetic and styling results that can be achieved with our hair once it has left the scalp can be enhanced if we clearly understand this principle and carefully apply the appropriate cosmetic science in its care.

In the past scientists and cosmetic formulators may have focused on the traditional hair 'types', and developed hair products on the basis of limited assumptions. Today's consumers worldwide are more sophisticated, and look more and more for 'end benefit' for *their* hair. The scientists' response to increasing awareness of hair diversity is the provision of increasing product diversity, to improve 'end benefit' results for every kind of hair.

Most people particularly as they grow older are looking for increased volume, and for volume control – the maintenance of sleek, smooth shining hair. Those with curly hair, which traditionally presents unique problems, seek ways of enabling them to manage it easily and care for it effectively. For those who have coloured hair, the first priority is to protect the colour. Others feel they above all need anti-dandruff or other speciality ingredients in the products they choose.

GROOMING

Grooming the hair is a regular habit in all primates. In most of our nearest relatives it is a social activity related to the removal of parasites and plant fragments, and is associated with bonding. In our more sophisticated society it can be either solitary or social (as at the hairdresser's).

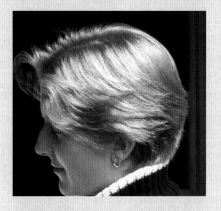

Well-groomed honey-blonde Nordic hair, its appearance repaying its owner's conscientious, regular care.

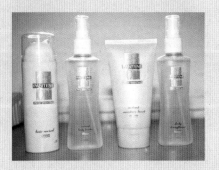

Scientists formulate specialised hair care products for every type of hair.

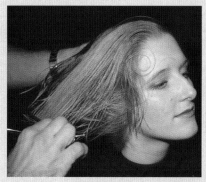

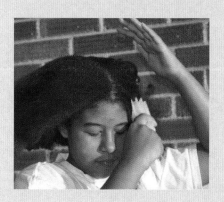

Gentle grooming prevents damage to the hair cuticle. Fine Indo-European hair may be easier to comb when wet, as less force is required. On the other hand grooming long African hair is difficult, wet or dry.

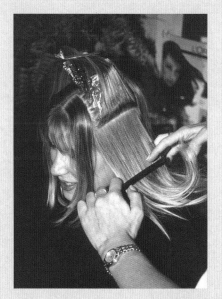

The services of a first-class stylist are invaluable. The cut is the starting point for all good hair care.

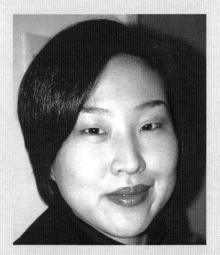

In the Orient many women wash their hair at night and let it dry naturally.

The ease with which hair can be groomed depends on the nature of the hair, its condition and the implements used. Straight wet hair requires less force to groom than dry hair does, since there is less friction between the comb and the hair. Curly hair, especially African-type hair, requires more force than straight hair and particularly so when it is dry: some published work indicates that a force more than 10 times greater is needed. If the protective cuticle is damaged, this leads ultimately to weathering.

WASHING HAIR

The aim of washing hair is to remove accumulated grease, sebum, dust, flakes of dead skin and pollutants. This depends on using hair care products that contain effective but mild **surfactant** systems (see page 53). These transform such substances into water-soluble forms so that they can be rinsed off the hair.

Whatever its nature, hair may be safely washed regularly provided that well-formulated hair care products are used. Tailoring cleansing systems to the individual need is the job of the cosmetic scientist. Factors that influence the process are associated with the length and quality of the hair shafts. The presence of hair shafts that have suffered cosmetic damage (often self-inflicted) may lead to a disappointing result if the wrong type of product is selected. Modern ranges of products are developed to accommodate this.

In practice, how the hair is washed depends on social and cultural factors, as does the frequency of washing—ranging from once or twice daily to never! In societies where water is scarce, frequent western-style shampooing and rinsing is impossible. Even in areas with plentiful water 'on tap', however, the density and length of hair may necessitate pre-soaking.

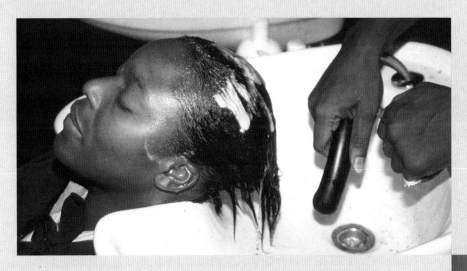

Washing 'African' hair is much easier if it has been relaxed. In its natural state it can be washed with an ordinary retail shampoo, but it presents more difficulty if worn long.

Washing long Indo-European or Oriental hair does not present any real problem. Washing short 'African' hair is also relatively easy, but washing long hair that is tightly curled may be much more difficult. Pre-soaking may be necessary to ensure the whole head is thoroughly wet, and the shampoo should be well worked into the scalp with the hands in order to ensure it reaches the roots of the hair. Many people with 'African' hair choose to reduce the frequency of shampooing, or keep their hair in a braided style for ease of management.

CONDITIONING

Conditioning after shampooing is an invaluable part of the regular hair care routine.

Conditioners (see pages 53-54) are designed to deposit a film of material on the hair shaft, especially at the edges of the cuticle scales and at any point where the cuticle is damaged. As a result the cuticle of conditioned hair lies flat and close to the cortex, so that a comb or brush passes through the hair with little friction or drag, and detangling is much easier. This is of particular

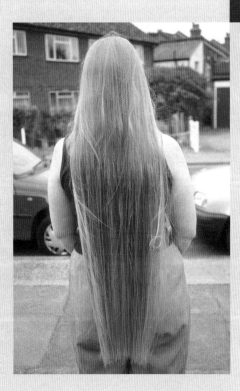

Washing long hair piled up on the head is potentially damaging, and if the hair is heavily weathered may result in tangling or even 'birds-nesting'.

Long, fine 'virgin' hair. Conditioning the ends will be necessary. Weathered hair will require intensive conditioning.

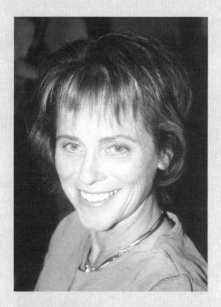

Fine hair cut into a modified bob with base brown colour and highlights; styling mousse and a flexible-hold spray increase the volume, and produce a dramatic change in hair appearance.

value on weathered or permed hair, since the conditioner protects the cuticle from further damage. The film also reduces the development of electric charges on the hair; these are the principal cause of 'fly-away' hair and can be troublesome in very dry environments. Conditioners leave the hair smooth, soft and manageable, with a good lustre.

CARING FOR FINE OR LONG HAIR

The diameter of fine hair may only be half that of coarse hair. Its form may be straight or wavy, but if worn long it tends to have little natural volume or 'body'.

Fine hair may be exceptionally difficult to style if left to grow much beyond shoulder length. In the very young this is seldom an aesthetic problem. Over time, however, and particularly from the teens onwards, the tip of the hair below the shoulder-blade may become very damaged (after all, this hair left the scalp five or six years earlier). Simply immersing it in water together with the regular use of hair dryers takes its toll on the hair, and the last few centimetres may show the classical signs of weathering (see page 51), including losing its shine.

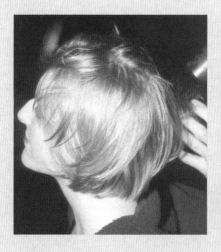

After expert layering, it is important that the hair is dried gently with the dryer well away from the head.

Styling tips for
fine hair

Start with a **good cut**

Use appropriate styling aids and products.
A **volumising shampoo, mousse** and **hair spray** can all help to give the hair more shape and body. **Waxes** and **gels** may remove volume but are effective in creating a style.

Avoid back-combing fine hair. Although it can give the appearance of volume by lifting, damage can ensue if the treatment is too vigorous or too frequent.

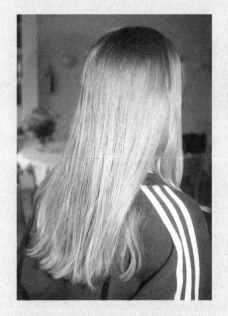 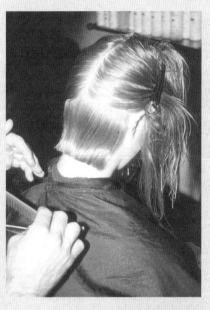 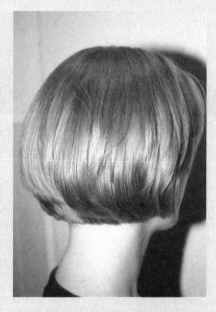

Without styling products, fine Nordic hair tends to hang limply unless given a layered cut ...

...here, a stylish bob is set with mousse to improve volume...

... the result!

Fine, low-density hair is best cut in layers, as this improves volume. The use of hair care products such as volumising shampoos, conditioners and mousses similarly improves the 'volume up' of hair.

CARING FOR OILY HAIR

There are two main reasons why oils may build up in the hair: either the sebum glands produce too much oil, or the amount of hair is insufficient to take up the normal quantity of oil produced. Perspiration from the head can also create greasy-looking strands, particularly in fine hair.

The degree of sebum production is determined partly by genetic inheritance and partly by the presence of male sex hormones (androgens) in both sexes. Androgen production by the body is at its peak in young men and women in their teens and twenties. Sebum production cannot be controlled without the use of oral drugs, but there is much that we can do to deal with the sebum itself once it is on the scalp.

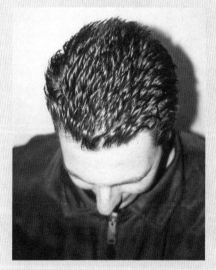

Excess sebum produces oily hair.

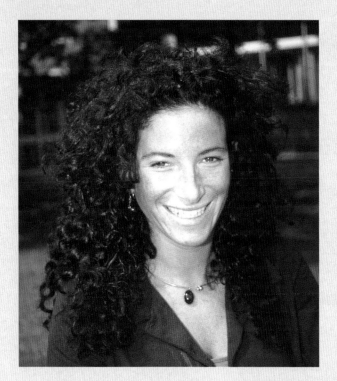

Beautiful dark curls proclaim this lady's Gypsy heritage. Gypsies are members of the original Indo-European peoples. Maintaining the beauty of such long hair requires hard work and care.

Hair that becomes oily quickly can be washed as often as time and economics allow. Shampooing once or even twice daily will do no harm, provided that appropriate conditioning is maintained. This will *not* in itself encourage sebum production.

Hair care products specially designed for oily hair should be selected. These can provide the desired end benefit since they will not contain excessive grease, wax or other substances that could worsen the oil deposition problem and make the hair style 'collapse' more quickly.

CARING FOR CURLY HAIR

Naturally curly hair often possesses the springiness that is missing in straight hair. On the one hand this can be viewed as something positive, because curly hair looks very 'vigorous'. On the other hand it can be difficult to maintain a style and to keep the curls well defined and looking healthy.

Natural curls can look particularly beautiful when they have a high gloss. This is often missing, however, not necessarily because of hair damage but because the wavy surface of curly hair does

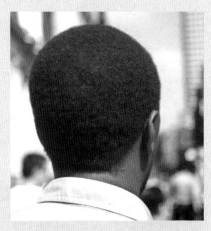

Curly African hair is easy to care for if it is kept short.

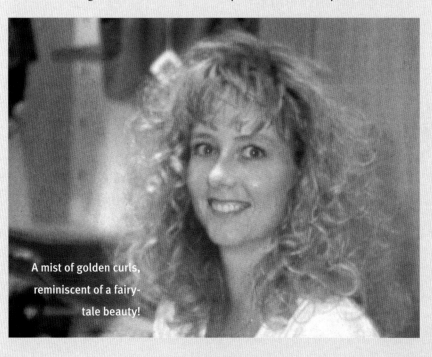

A mist of golden curls, reminiscent of a fairy-tale beauty!

not reflect the light as well as does smooth, straight hair. More shine can be achieved on curly hair by using products formulated with reflectant oils.

CARING FOR WEATHERED HAIR

Any type of hair – fine, coarse or woolly – can be damaged by weathering. The finer or flatter the hair, the less effort is required to damage it. Perming is especially harmful to fine hair, as is heat to 'African' hair, and repeated bleaching can damage even the normally resistant Oriental hair.

In weathered hair it is the hair shaft that has been damaged: damage may be local, focal or extensive. In the process of weathering the cuticle becomes worn down and the cortex may be partly or significantly exposed. Its physical characteristics may gradually change: it tends to have increased porosity, diminished texture and reduced elasticity, and it feels dry, rough and brittle. Weathered hair has less shine, and it may be difficult to style. Gross rupture of the cortex may be seen as 'split ends', especially if the hair is worn long. The causes of weathering may be one or more of the following:

- poor-quality daily care
- repeated or excessive back-combing, which tends to roughen and damage the hair surface
- using heated rollers or curlers too often or too hot: dry heat draws moisture out of the hair and makes it brittle
- gross over-exposure to the sun – long periods of sunbathing need to be followed by thorough conditioning
- severe perming or relaxing procedures, especially when carried out inexpertly
- the use of poorly formulated hair colouring materials or bleaches
- long periods of growth.

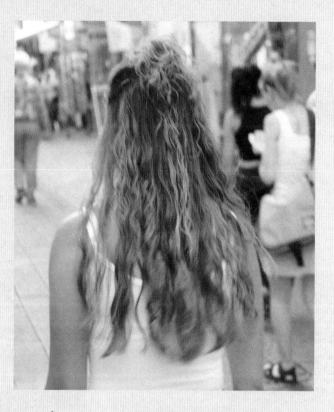

Badly weathered coloured hair, needing intensive conditioning

This frequently coloured, dry hair needs special protection and conditioning.

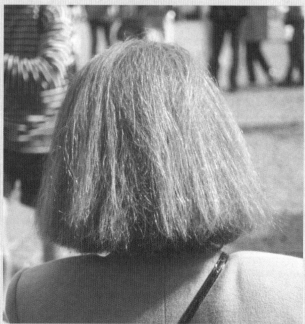

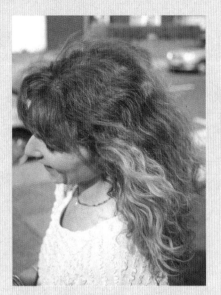

This lady used to have her hair bleached but is now growing it out. Regular intensive conditioning is essential.

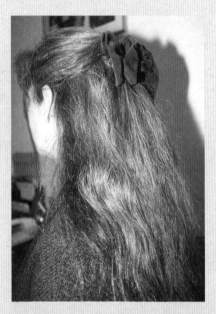

Long hair with a high percentage of grey in a lady of 65. Unfortunately, hair quality naturally declines with age; a shorter style might show better results.

Weathering in long hair

Because of its age, long hair may have experienced a substantial amount of exposure to the sun and to cosmetic treatment. This shows itself particularly in the lower third of the hair. There are often significant structural differences between healthy roots and worn ends. It is very important that hair is not allowed to grow unchecked; the ends should be trimmed regularly and expertly.

Preventing weathering

Severely weathered hair cannot be cured, only cut off, but much can be done in the way of prevention.

When washing hair, it is essential to use high-quality shampoos and conditioners and to choose types that are appropriate to the hair.

Regular intensive conditioning (see pages 47-48) will reduce the grooming friction, and will improve hydration and minimise porosity.

Preparations for brittle, split hair often bear on their labels the technical term 'active polymer'. These polymers are synthetic substances with large molecules. The keratin of damaged hair draws such substances to itself like a magnet, and they coat and protect the hair. Re-hydration and improved shine may result, although the effects are usually only temporary.

Silk proteins and collagens are both found in treatments for weathered hair, and also bind closely to the hair. Panthenol, which is a derivative of the vitamin B complex, is also useful: it helps to provide more moisture and elasticity to the cortex. Fine oils such as wheatgerm or jojoba oil gently film over the hair and make it more flexible.

HAIR CARE PRODUCTS

For many years, and often even today, specially formulated hair care products have been marketed for hair that was 'normal', 'dry/permed/damaged' or 'greasy'. This reflects an approach based on an understanding of the physiology of the hair shaft. In the future it may be that this understanding is translated into the technologies that correct abnormal physiology and confer 'end benefit' on the user.

Shampoos

Worldwide, the most commonly used hair care product is a cleanser. For most of the first world this is an aqueous mixture containing mild surfactants (see below) – a shampoo. Early shampoos were products designed simply to remove sebum, perspiration, dirt and dead cells shed from the skin. They have now been transformed into agents that not only cleanse but also beautify and add volume to the hair.

Soap shampoo was the original hair cleanser, and in parts of the developing world bar soaps derived from wood ash are still used today. Soaps consist simply of sodium salts of fatty acids plus oils. Their advantages were their cleansing properties and cheapness. The major drawbacks were their harshness and the fact that they form an unpleasant scum in hard water. Since hard water is so widespread, soap shampoos are seldom used today by choice.

New shampoo formulations based on sulphonated oils started to become popular in the 1950s. These contain **surfactants** (often called **detergents**) for their cleansing and foaming power, together with secondary ingredients to improve and condition the hair. The surfactants have a twofold action: part of the surfactant molecule removes the dirt from the hair and part transfers it to the rinse water. Many modern well-formulated shampoos also contain conditioning agents (see below), to improve the manageability and shine of the hair.

Some shampoos are described as being specially formulated for different hair types. A shampoo formulated for oily hair generally contains stronger surfactants and a lower proportion of conditioner. A shampoo for dry hair usually contains milder surfactants, though they are less effective cleansers. Shampoos for limp or fine hair contain less conditioner, because conditioners are designed to reduce curling and fluffing, but they may contain protein additives to give the hair extra body. Permed or damaged hair needs surfactants of the very mildest kind.

Conditioners

Most modern conditioners are emulsions of oils or waxes in water, and many contain silicones such as dimethicone and care-

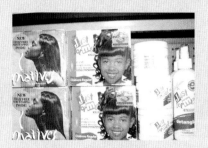

Certain products are formulated especially for specific cultures.

The frizz in this hair might have been prevented by thorough conditioning as well as by a good cut.

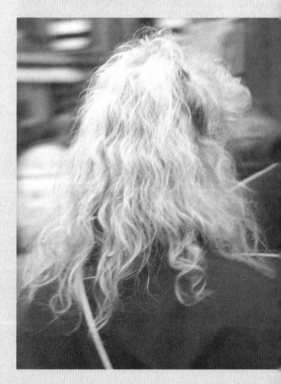

Styling mousse helps to create and
hold the desired effect.

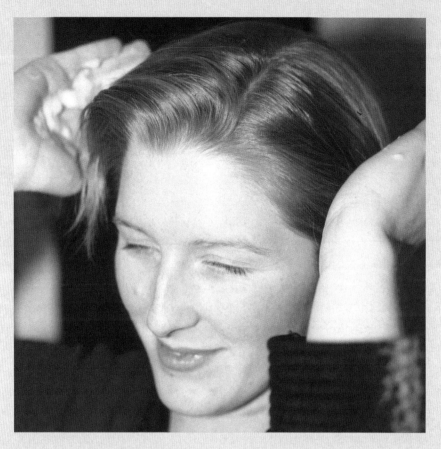

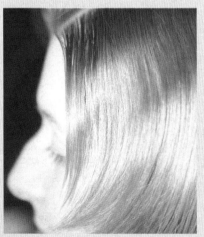

... the result!

fully designed polymers. Modern conditioners prevent the hair
from becoming lank, and come in various types of formulation:

- 'regular' conditioners are applied to the hair after each
  shampoo; most are rinsed out immediately, but some can be
  left on the hair
- special products are available for frequent use
- intensive conditioners, often cream formulations, are applied
  once or twice a week and left on for several hours; these are
  especially useful for dry or weathered hair
- portable spray conditioners are for use as a quick fix to
  temporarily improve the appearance of weathered hair and
  split ends
- some products contain UV filters to protect hair colour.

Oils and pomades

Heavy **emollients** and **oils** have long been used to assist in grooming hair. In the developing world, castor oil and mineral oils are
still widely used for African hair.

Pomades consist mainly of petrolatum, lanolin, mineral oil and olive oil, together with perfume. Solid **brilliantines** are composed of vegetable or mineral oils with waxes, sometimes together with vitamin supplements and plant oils such as aloe vera. These agents coat the hair, reducing the static electric charges between the hairs and making it easier to comb.

Products like these keep the hair in place by literally plastering it down. This results in some plasticisation of the keratin in the hair shaft, which makes the hair – especially 'African' hair – more manageable.

Moisturisers

Moisturisers contain humectants that attract water to the keratin fibres and hold it there. Very dry hair, and especially 'African' hair, can be combed more easily if it is kept adequately moisturised. Hair that has been chemically curled or waved will require more moisturising than untreated hair. Most of the popular moisturisers on the market contain lanolin or its derivatives. Glycerin in significant concentrations (20 to 50%) and propylene glycol are excellent moisturisers that carry little risk of causing irritation. They are less suitable for hair that has been treated with chemical relaxers or a hot comb, because they tend to make relaxed hair look lank and the hot-pressed hair may revert to its pre-processed state.

Modern retail hair care products are designed for consumers worldwide. 'African' hair can be protected and moisturised by conditioning agents that are often perceived as being suitable only for Indo-European and Oriental hair.

Styling aids

Styling gels and waxes create a thick, tacky gel that dries on the hair, leaving it stiff and fixed in the preferred style hair. Mousses also help styling, but are soft to feel and are easily removed. Hair sprays are useful aids to maintaining volume.

Activators

Activators are products specifically designed for curls. They contain certain proteins and/or plant oils (soybean or wheat germ oil), which cause the curl pattern to tighten.

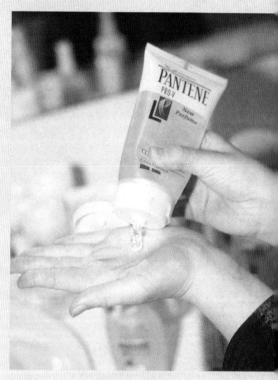

Styling gel is popular among young people of all regions.

Modern hair sprays do not gum the hair together into rigid masses, but produce flexible 'spot welds' to hold it in a gentle style.

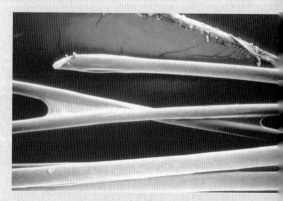

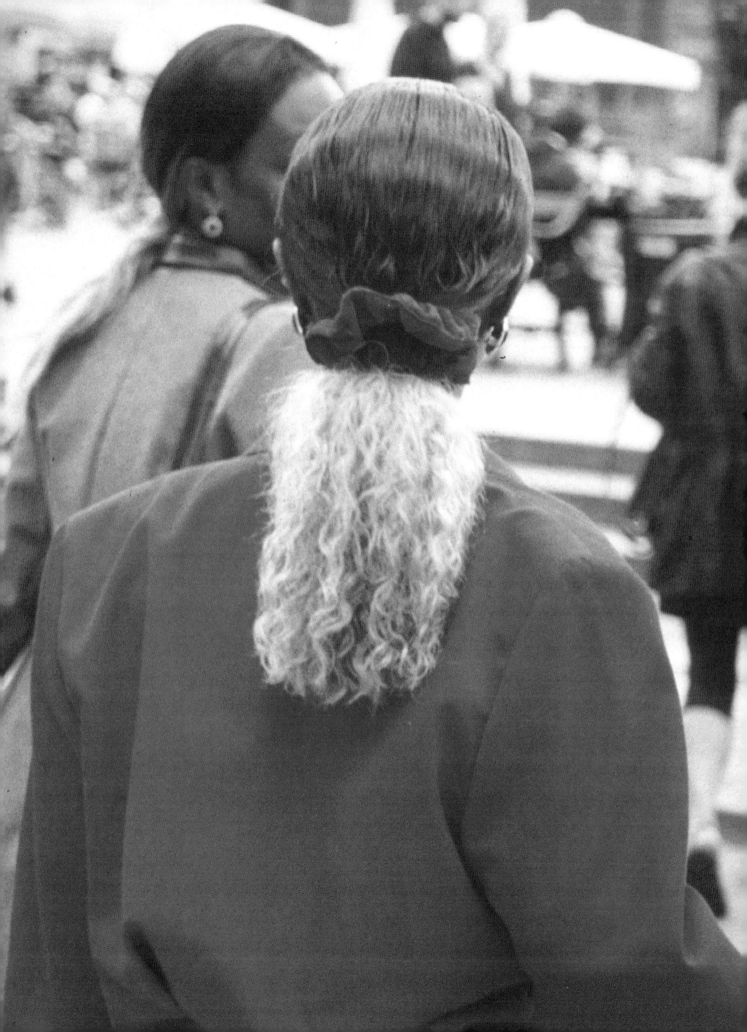

CHAPTER 7
Hair Diversity and Hair Treatments

Whatever the nature of the hair shaft, physical and chemical treatments can help to change style, make hair more manageable, add volume and make it possible to alter its original properties temporarily or even permanently. Repeated or excessive 'permanent' changes, however, can diminish the fundamental quality of the hair and result in damage or breakage.

SETTING

Setting is a relatively simple way of transforming the appearance of the hair. Whenever the hair is washed, contact with water breaks the weak hydrogen bonds between the protein chains. These bonds are partially responsible for the form of the hair shaft. Damp, softened straight hair can be rearranged into a preferred shape (often on rollers), perhaps a curl or wave, and gently dried. As it dries, the hydrogen bonds re-form in new positions and hold it in its altered arrangement. (Further contact with water, even atmospheric moisture, causes the bonds to revert to their old positions, however.) Conversely, curly hair may be temporarily smoothed and straightened by the same process. Finally, application of hair spray 'sets' the creation.

HOT-COMBING

Hot-combing, also known as **hair-pressing**, is still common among people with curly African hair. An emollient such as petrolatum is applied to the hair, and this is followed by combing with a hot metal comb – the temperature may exceed 400°F. The treated hair remains straight until moisture causes reversion by restoring the hydrogen bonds to their original positions. Pomades (see

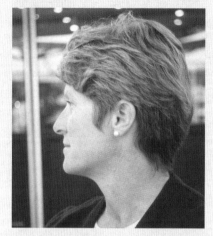

After applying mousse and blow-drying, setting the hair with flexible hair spray creates 'volume up'.

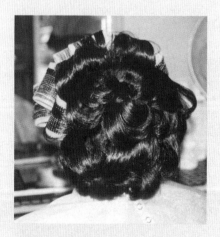

Relaxed 'African' hair can be set in the same manner as Indo-European hair, giving greater styling potential.

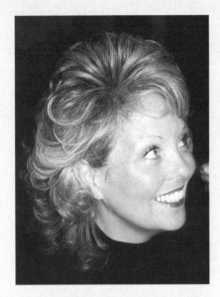

Perming increases volume, but
afterwards the hair needs special
attention to reduce dryness.

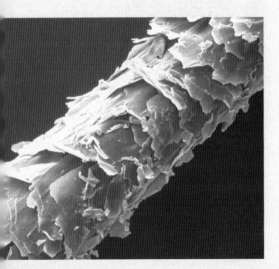

Seriously over-treated hair; no wonder
it looks dry, rough and dull.

page 55) are often used to prevent this reversion and to add
sheen.

This use of rollers or hot curling irons can accelerate 'weathering' of the hair, and can even inflict scalp burns. There is also a
danger of **hot-comb alopecia**, due to damage to the hair follicle.
This condition is characterised by a well-defined area of partial
hair loss over the top of the head, presumably though not certainly as a result of the hot petrolatum running down the hair
shaft and on to the scalp.

PERMING

Chemical **perming** is part of diverse hair care and is present to a
greater or lesser degree in all cultures. It waxes and wanes in fashion, and when performed correctly it may be a useful method of
increasing volume. In later life hair density and hair length naturally decline, and it is very frequently used by older people.

In perming, in contrast to setting, it is the strong disulphide
bonds of the hair cortex that are changed. The initial breakdown
(reduction) is brought about by the application of perming solution (usually based on thioglycollic acid or a related compound),
which opens the scale of the cuticle, softens the hair and allows
the solution to enter the cortex. The hair can be rearranged over
rollers as required for the formation of waves or curls, and then
treated with a neutralising solution (oxidation). This causes the
disulphide bonds to form in their new positions and permanently
to lock the hair into its altered shape. The treated portion will
keep this shape as new hair grows out (unless it is re-permed,
which is a damaging procedure that should be embarked upon
with caution). Important differences between perming solutions
include:

• the strength – how much of the active chemical is present: this
  varies considerably and affects the process speed
• the pH, that is, the degree of alkalinity; the higher the
  alkalinity, the stronger the product
• the contact time (length of processing) required.

Hair is always to some extent damaged by perming, however
carefully it is done, and special care is needed thereafter. Because
of its increased porosity it should not be washed for some days
after being processed, and when a normal washing routine begins

a special shampoo for permed or damaged hair should always be used. Regular conditioning is advisable.

RELAXING PROCESSES

Relaxing hair is a process of removing curl or wave, wholly or in part. The process is the direct reverse of perming, designed for people with naturally very curly hair who want it looser, softly curled or straight. Many women with African hair are unable to achieve any length in their hair style until their hair has been relaxed.

Most early relaxing processes were physically based and temporary in their effects, but today's chemical techniques can produce effective and permanent results in the hands of experts. Hair type (curly or wavy) and hair texture (fine, medium or coarse) are factors to consider when taking decisions as to which relaxer to use, and in what concentration, and how long it should be left on the hair. 'Virgin' hair (hair that has never been chemically treated) may be particularly resistant to relaxing.

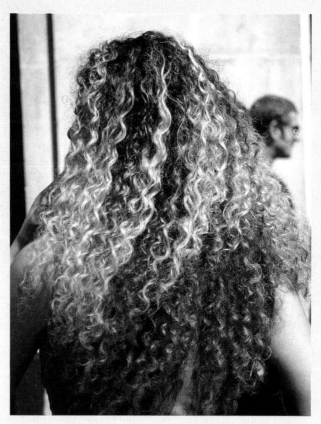

Perming and bleaching add style, but for long hair subsequent care is particularly important.

The permanent methods involve the use of chemical relaxers. Those available at the time of writing include:
- ammonium thioglycollate-based lotions made for looser-curled hair, such as European-type hair
- ammonium thioglycollate-based creams intended specifically for African-type hair
- creams or gels based on sodium hydroxide (caustic soda or 'lye'), made for Afro-Caribbean hair
- creams or gels based on calcium hydroxide and guanidine hydroxide, called 'non-lye products', made for tightly curled hair and a wide range of hair textures
- creams based on ammonium and sodium bisulphites.

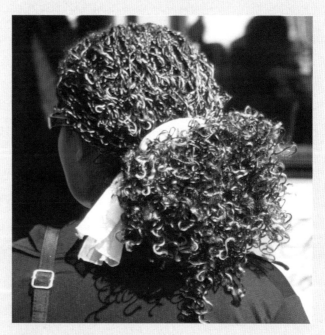

A long semi-relaxed 'Afro'.

African hair presents management problems; relaxing will help.

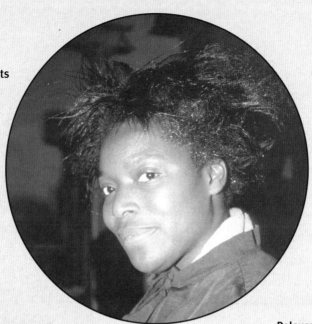

Relaxer being applied to the roots of the hair...

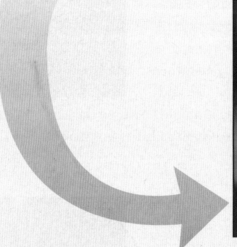

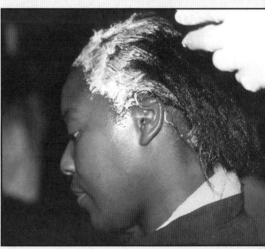

The treatment was carried out at the Terry Jacques Salon, Clapham.

The client is a 25-year-old lady from central Africa with tight curls, which are to be relaxed and styled to straighten.

relaxing
& styling

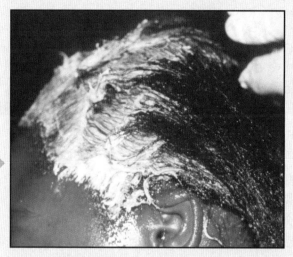

... and is well worked in ...

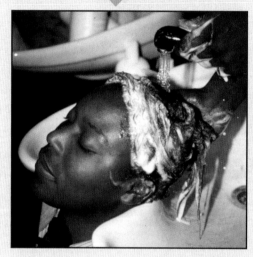

... before being rinsed off.

The smoothed relaxed hair
is oiled and pomaded to
improve control.

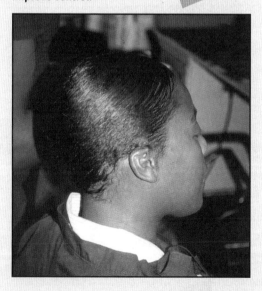

Relaxation completed:
a pleasing and
attractive result.

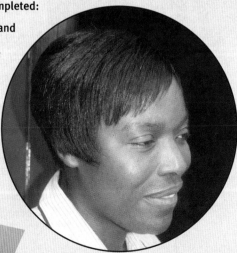

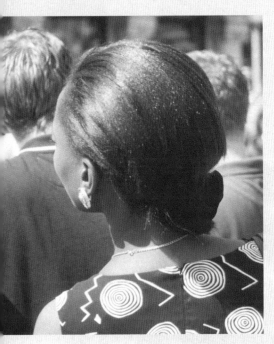

Relaxed hair needs special attention.
Smoothing gels can help.

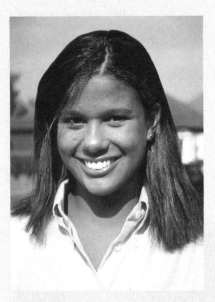

Relaxed hair in a girl whose hair shows
both Indo-European and African
characteristics.

Two types of relaxer are especially popular: sodium hydroxide relaxers (potassium hydroxide and lithium hydroxide relaxers are also available and work similarly) and guanidine hydroxide relaxers. The last-named have become increasingly widely used by professional hair stylists and are less caustic than the other relaxers. Guanidine hydroxide itself is an unstable organic base, and has to be prepared by mixing calcium hydroxide base with guanidine carbonate solution before application to the hair.

Relaxing with a thioglycollate derivative is a two-step process, similar to permanent waving. Relaxers based on alkali (either sodium hydroxide or guanidine hydroxide) depend on rather different chemistry. The alkali breaks down the disulphide bonds in hair by hydrolysis – that is, the breakdown of a substance by, and with, water. The hair softens and relaxes, tight curls are loosened, and the hair can be moulded into a more relaxed shape. When a sufficient degree of relaxation is reached the hair is washed with an acid-balancing shampoo, which returns it to its normal acid state. No oxidising neutraliser is used: the chemical process consists of the single hydrolysis step.

Some products require that adequate basing – the application of protective gels or creams to the skin around the hairline and ears – is made before the relaxing process begins.

Whichever relaxer is used, it is important to vet closely the subsequent use of other chemical processes on the relaxed hair because the basic nature of the hair has been changed. Fewer disulphide bridges are now present, so further reduction processes should never be used.

'Curling' relaxed hair

Once relaxed, the straightened hair offers greater opportunity for styling and can now be re-permed, waved or curled in the same way as Indo-European hair.

The curl or wave process is a two-step procedure requiring that any chemically unaltered new growth be straightened first and set on rollers. The steps are based on thioglycollate-based products. After rinsing, the hair is saturated with an oxidising agent (neutraliser), usually sodium bromate. The second and third steps of this process are essentially identical to perming.

Curling and waving, like relaxation, can cause severe hair breakage, but the breakage will usually be more widespread and limited to the ends of the hair shafts. With curls and waves, the entire hair shaft is treated with the thioglycollate each time the hair is redone, which can lead to serious hair shaft damage.

Problems with hair relaxation

Mild caustic burns of the scalp and neck after relaxation are sometimes experienced with the alkali relaxers. More severe burns, even resulting in blistering, occur occasionally, but scarring and permanent hair loss are rare when relaxation is carried out by an expert. Any skin inflammation that occurs may be followed by the appearance of pigmented markings that may last some time.

BLEACHING AND COLOURING

Since ancient times peoples of all cultures have chosen to change or modify their hair colour. This change may be part of a fashion trend, a social statement, or just to create a temporary or perma-

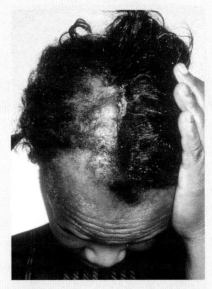

Scalp burn from inexpert relaxing.

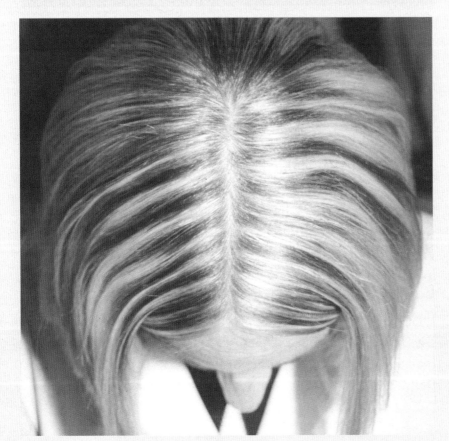

Cleverly alternating patterns of colour. The hair is in good condition after regular use of hair care products

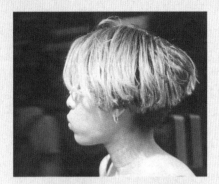

Colouring relaxed African hair may profoundly affect the hair shaft.

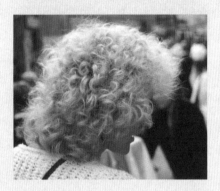

Dry bleached hair, desperately in need of conditioning.

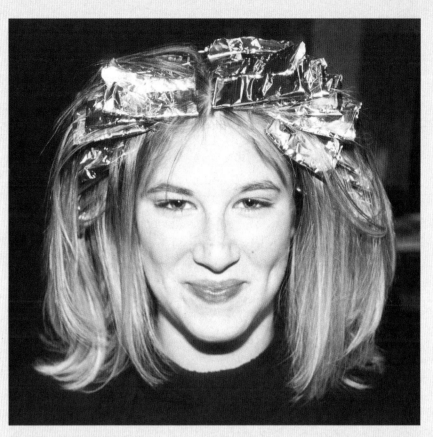

Highlights being added to hair by a top salon; these add flair and style, and are in keeping with skin colour.

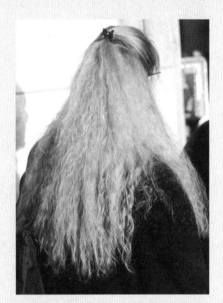

Use of a single dramatic colour creates a stark effect, which may not reflect nature!

nent change in their 'image'. Bleaching dark hair, as well as further lightening blonde hair, is very common. The addition of colour, particularly red, is widespread, and henna dye is still used for this purpose in eastern countries.

Throughout the world, the single most common reason for colouring the hair is the wish to disguise unwanted **grey hairs**. Grey hair is caused by the reduction, or the almost complete cessation, of pigment production in the hair follicle. This is probably under genetic control and to a greater or lesser extent this colour loss will affect us all sooner or later. No hair type is immune. Sometimes the unpigmented hairs may be coarser in texture than their neighbours on the scalp, and many find their greying hair is dryer and less lustrous than it used to be. Covering grey was originally carried out using salts of heavy metals such as lead. Modern well-formulated products contain safe synthetic dyes.

Bleaching partially or wholly destroys pigments in the hair shaft, whether they are the natural pigments (melanins) or pigments remaining from previous colouring treatments. Hydrogen peroxide solution is invariably used as the bleaching chemical: the strength of the solution used depends on the final hair shade required. Complete destruction of melanin requires a relatively strong solution, and leads to hair that is almost white (not a pure white, since keratin itself has a very pale yellow colour). Partial removal of melanin gives brown, reddish or yellowish hair, depending on the initial shade of the hair and the strength of the bleach. Often just a part of the hair is lightened, to give a 'highlighted' effect.

If a complete and permanent change of colour is required (and today's consumer can choose virtually any shade), the hair is often bleached first to remove the existing pigment; alternatively the dye may be mixed with hydrogen peroxide. In both cases the effect is to open the cuticle scales enough for the dye molecules to pass through into the cortex, where they are oxidised into larger, intensely coloured particles that are unable to pass out of the hair and remain there until the hair grows out.

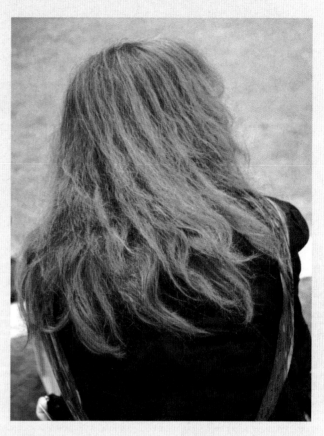

Home hair colouring can result in very weathered hair unless good hair care is exercised

Both bleaching and colouring increase the porosity and reduce the elasticity of the hair, which hence needs great care and attention thereafter. Very rarely, a treatment results in catastrophe. You can minimise *your* risk by understanding the nature and diversity of hair, consulting with professionals and using high-quality products – which is, after all, everyone's recipe for great hair!

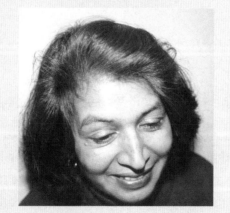

Henna has been used for centuries to colour the hair.

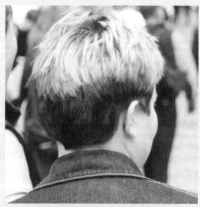

Modern colour makes a statement!

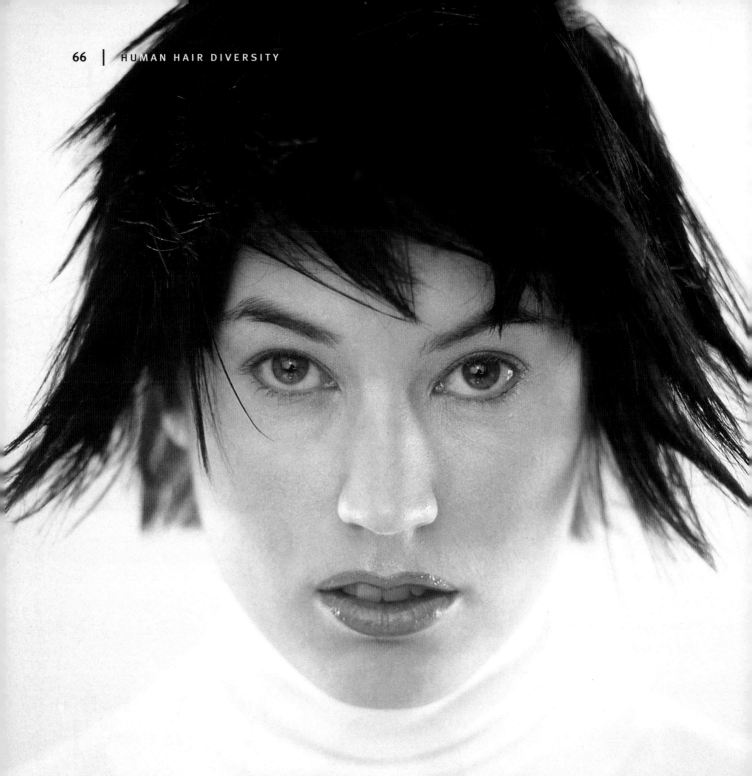

We hope you have enjoyed reading this book on
human hair diversity.

We are indeed all part of one species and as we become more
homogeneous as a society we may see even greater diversity of
our single most evident characteristic: our hair.

Care of this unique asset is our joint concern.

Glossary

alopecia: loss of hair (as in male and female pattern androgenetic alopecia)

bottlenecking: reduction of the genetic heterogeneity of a population by a drastic decrease in numbers, e.g. by famine, catastrophe or geographical isolation

cline: continuous variation in form between members of a species with a wide variable geographical or ecological range

common ancestor: an individual (or group) from whom the individuals (or groups) in question are all descended directly

emollient: substance that has a softening or soothing effect on the skin

evolution: gradual change of characteristics of a population over successive generations; accounts for the origin of new species

gene: the biological unit of heredity, each consisting of a short length of DNA; the genes in any individual are a combination of genes derived from the organism's parents. A human cell may contain more than 100,000 genes (the exact number is currently hotly debated), arranged long chromosomes. Genes carry the specification for the manufacture of proteins and hence determine each organism's individual characteristics, including (in humans) hair type and colour.

genotype: the genetic constitution of an organism

humectant: a substance used to reduce loss of moisture

lineage: a line of direct descendants from an ancestor

micron: a unit of length equal to one-millionth of a metre (10^{-6} m)

natural selection: process resulting in the survival of those individuals in a population that are best adapted to the prevailing conditions

pH: measure of acidity or alkalinity

population: all the members of a particular species, e.g. humans, in a particular area

primates: the group of animals that comprises creatures such as apes, monkeys and humans; characterised by flexible hands with opposable thumbs, good eyesight and relatively large brains

proteins: organic compounds with a very large molecule composed of long chains of amino acid units; proteins are vital constituents of all living cells

sebum: fatty secretions from the sebaceous glands, which are associated with terminal hairs

set: a group of peoples having certain features or characteristics in common

silicones: highly stable compounds consisting of chains of silicon and oxygen atoms, with a wide range of applications – their incorporation into hair care products was justifiably described as a technological breakthrough

surfactants: substances that can reduce the surface tension of water

virgin hair: hair that has never had any physical or chemical treatment

Index